TOUCH ME PLEASE

Second Book in the Series

LOVE ME, TOUCH ME, HEAL ME

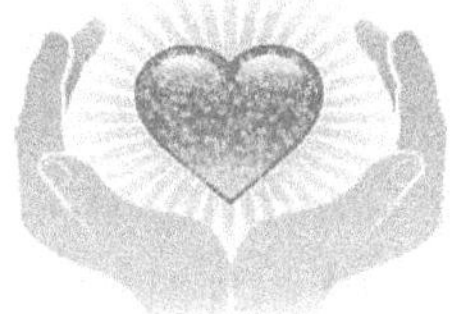

THE PATH TO

* PHYSICAL
* EMOTIONAL
* SEXUAL
* SPIRITUAL

REAWAKENING

Dr. Erica Goodstone

Touch Me … Please, Book II, is dedicated to

- **My teacher and mentor, Ilana Rubenfeld, whose gentle yet powerful training which combined talk with touch, The Rubenfeld Synergy Method, set the course for my life's work.**
- **Dr. Seena Russell, for mentoring me in both Rubenfeld Synergy and spiritual centeredness**
- **Waturo Oshashi, who taught me the meaning and depth of shiatsu meridians, energy, physical and emotional anatomy and healing**
- **Dr. John Upledger, for teaching me that only 5 ounces of touch can be more powerful and curative than any amount of deep and painful pressure**
- **Dr. John Beaulieu, for mentoring and guiding me in the use of sound, vibration, color, observation, Eriksonian hypnosis, and Dr. Randolph Stone's comprehensively holistic Polarity Therapy Method**
- **Dr. Tiffany Field, for creating a massive amount of research revealing and corroborating the healing potential of massage and body therapies**
- **Dr. Candace Pert, for her ground breaking research about the way neurotransmitters spread throughout the body, in her book, _Molecules of Emotion_**

Publisher Data & Legal Information

ISBN: 978-0-9824304-5-3

Published by Create Healing and Love Now Publishers

Contact the Publisher at RelationshipHealingToolbox.com

Every attempt has been made by the author to provide acknowledgement of the sources used for the material in this book. If there has been an omission of any source, please contact the author at DrErica@DrEricaWellness.com.

Disclaimer: No responsibility is assumed by the authors/publishers for any injury and/or damage and/or loss sustained in persons or property as a result of using this product; and/or for any liability, negligence or otherwise use or operation of any products, methods, instructions or ideas contained in the material herein.

The views and opinions expressed in this book and related materials are derived from the author's experience and research as a professor of health and physical education, yoga and meditation teacher, licensed mental health counselor, licensed professional counselor, licensed marriage and family therapist, board certified sex therapist, licensed massage and bodywork therapist, certified pain management practitioner, certified Integrative Medicine practitioner, certified Polarity Therapist, certified Rubenfeld Synergist, and involvement with numerous professional associations. She is not a licensed M.D. and does not diagnose or claim to cure any physical disease. She is also not a psychiatrist and does not claim to cure mental illness.

Any reader currently under the care or supervision of a psychiatrist, physician or other medical or behavioral health practitioner is urged to seek their professional advice before using or practicing any of the material or techniques contained herein.

ABOUT THE AUTHOR

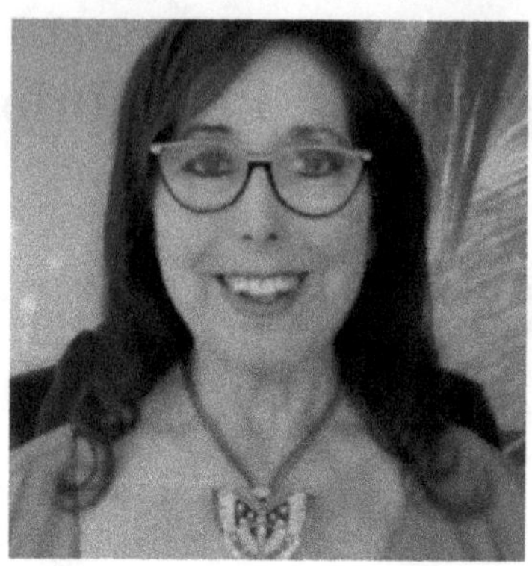

Erica Goodstone, Ph.D., has devoted her life's work to the discovery of love, healing and the creation of intimate, satisfying, fulfilling and joyful relationships. During over two decades, through her lectures, seminars and private counseling sessions, she has worked with thousands of men and women to create love and healing in their lives.

Having studied extensively from many different sources, Dr. Goodstone is a licensed mental health counselor, professional counselor, marriage and family therapist, massage and bodywork therapist. She is a diplomate and fellow for the American Association of Integrative Medicine and a diplomate for the American Academy of Pain Management. Dr. Goodstone is also a diplomate for the American Board of Sexology, a fellow for the American Academy of Clinical Sexologists, and a certified Sex Therapist for the American Association of Sexuality Educators and Therapists.

As a former professor of health and physical education at F.I.T./State University of New York, Dr. Goodstone spent 25 years studying and teaching about the body: physical fitness, health and wellness, stress management, sports psychology, team building and human sexuality. But she did not stop there.

Dr. Goodstone also spent many years studying a wide variety of healing body therapy modalities in including massage, shiatsu, polarity therapy, craniosacral therapy, Reiki, reflexology, Chinese medical theory, Japanese healing theories. Her studies led to the combination of touch with counseling through the gentle yet profound Rubenfeld Synergy

Method. In fact, she was on the original steering committee and the board of directors for the first two terms of the U.S. Association for Body Psychotherapy. This was the first organization to bring together all the different originators and practitioners of somatic body psychotherapy methods and modalities.

But Dr. Goodstone's knowledge and background does not stop there. She has also fervently and passionately craved her own inner spiritual development and outer social awareness. Her seeking led her to spend many years studying yoga, first with the Sivananda Center in New York City and at the Sivananda Ashram in Paradise Island, Bahamas, where she met Swami Vishnu Devananda and listened to Ravi Shankar play the sitar. Later she spent years working with Guru Mayi, Swami Muktananda's disciple, receiving Darshan and personl counseling as needed.

Her studies included attending many consciousness raising seminars in the 1980's, including the EST seminars led by Werner Erhard, the Living Love Workshops led by Ken Keyes, Jr., author of *The Handbook to Higher Consciousness,* and DMA seminars about the creative process and structural thinking led by Robert Fritz.
She avidly studied the Rosicrucian manuals for many years, along with the Kaballah teachings of The Builders of the Adytum and the Course in Miracles. Her current focus has been exclusively upon the works of Joel Goldsmith, *The Infinite Way, and Siddha Yoga* Master Swami Muktananda..

Dr. Erica Goodstone has been a celebrated speaker at national and local professional and public events. Since her doctoral dissertation, which studied the effects of early mother-infant bonding upon later adult intimacy, she has continued to write extensively about creating love through the healing power of touch, intimacy, and the mind/body/spirit connection.

Dr. Goodstone's interviews and articles have appeared in *Who's Who of Medicine and Healthcare, CBS 4 TV, Blog Talk Radio Logical Soul Talk, Mademoiselle, Cosmopolitan , Marie Claire, Penthouse Forum, Journal of Sex and Marital therapy, Newsletters of the U.S. Association for Body Psychotherapy.* Dr. Goodstone has a very wide presence on the web. Her bio and blogs appear on numerous sites, e.g., Wordpress.com and Gather.com, as well as numerous ezines, most notably ezinearticles.com.

Dr. Goodstone's chapter, "Sexual Reawakening appears in the wonderfully organized book of Rubenfeld Synergy practitioners, *Healing Journeys: The Power of Rubenfeld Synergy, V. Mechner, Ed.* She has also written a section about touch therapies in the internationally acclaimed book, *The Continuum Complete International Encyclopedia of Sexuality*, R. J Noonan and R. Francoeur, Eds.

Dr. Goodstone can be reached at

DrErica@DrEricaWellness.com

****

INTRODUCTION TO THIS BOOK SERIES

Love Me, Touch Me, Heal Me: The Path to Physical, Emotional, Sexual and Spiritual Reawakening shows us what it takes to love, touch, and heal our own self. As we heal, we develop a renewed passion for life, a deep sense of being connected to something beyond our immediate life circumstances, and an increased desire for intimate loving. ***Love Me, Touch Me, Heal Me*** is meant to be a coming out party, coming out of hiding, bringing our total self into the light for examination, acceptance, and readiness to share our authentic self intimately with others.

Clients, colleagues and friends have often asked me to recommend a good book about love and relationships or about emotional intimacy and sexual communication. Others have requested information about ways to heal their body through natural methods, e.g., diet, exercise, body therapy, or even spirituality. And some have wondered what the best psychological approach might be to overcome fears, anxiety, anger, depression or relationship conflicts.

Answers to the above questions will be easily obtained as you read through this series of four ebooks. You will discover that you can find the answers to most of your problems, dilemmas, life issues and concerns through self-evaluation. As you complete the exercises, you will literally begin to heal your cellular memories, create new brain patterns and remove lifelong blocks to intimate joyful relating. You can turn to professionals for expert opinions, guidance, support and mentoring, but with this book you will begin to more fully trust your own inner knowing about what is truly best for your growth and healing.

FORMAT OF THIS BOOK

This **Book Series** is divided into four books consisting of three chapters in each book as follows:

Book I **Love Me … Please**

Chapter 1 **The Gift of Love**
Chapter 2 **Be Who You Are…The Greatest Gift of All**
Chapter 3 **The Delicate Dance of Love**

Book II **Touch Me … Please**

Chapter 1 **Your Body Believes You**
Chapter 2 **It's a Sensational World**
Chapter 3 **Touching Matters…The Profound Effects of Body Therapy**

Book III Heal Me … Please

Chapter 1 Heal Me…Please
Chapter 2 Let All Your Senses Speak…As You Heal
Chapter 3 Touching Stories…Healing Through Body Psychotherapy

Book IV Sexual and Spiritual Reawakening

Chapter 1 Ordinary People, Ordinary Yet Extraordinary Sex
Chapter 2 Ten Simple Steps to Sexual Reawakening
Chapter 3 Sexual And Spiritual Reawakening…At Last

- Every chapter contains vital information, theories, concepts and suggestions gleaned from years of study, research, personal and professional experiences.
- Every chapter includes pertinent real-life stories, individual and partner written, verbal and contemplative exercises.
- Every chapter builds upon the previous one in the healing process.
- Every chapter is also complete unto itself.
- You may choose to read one entire book from start to finish and then begin a second book.
- You may choose to start with a specific chapter in any of the books.

- Resources, references, and keywords will appear at the end of each book.

This entire series of four books was originally intended to be one book. Written many years ago, this book has been hibernating in file boxes until now, a time when this world needs all the love we can muster. And this book teaches us how.

Love Me, Touch Me, Heal Me: The Path to Physical, Emotional, Sexual and Spiritual Reawakening belongs in the personal library of anyone who truly wants to heal from the past and create loving, touching and authentically intimate relationships. This is a guidebook, a reference book, and a comforting friend along the path to reawakening.

HOW TO USE THIS BOOK

This book is about your life, my life, and all of our lives. Read this book, follow the exercises, and watch miracles happen. *Love Me, Touch Me, Heal Me* is a life transforming healing process. For best results, you will need a few basic materials.

1. ***Writing Materials***

a. **A journal, preferably a beautiful, special journal, but any 4" by 6" or 8" by 10" lined or unlined, notebook will do.** Choosing a journal or notebook that is special to you creates an experience of sensory stimulation every time you write in it! If you choose to write all the exercises in this book on pieces of paper, that's okay. But, if the outer appearance is appealing and soothing to your eyes, if the texture satisfies your sense of touch, if there's a fragrance of fresh cut paper or soft smooth leather that comforts you, the power of the words you write will be enhanced. Your brain will connect the sensual beauty of your journal with your written words and with your life. Your mind and body will begin to believe that you are serious about creating healing, love, spiritual connection, sexual aliveness, and joy in your life.

b. **Pen, pencil, colored pencils or crayons.** Brain research indicates that the mind absorbs information best when all the senses are involved. So get yourself a box of colored pencils, colored pens or crayons. You'll probably discover that you want some pastels, and maybe even paint and brushes before you're through. Colors and textures add additional dimensionality to your writing, increasing the possibility for your brain to record and store your hopes and dreams, uplifting words, goals, new beliefs, and appropriate affirmations. This allows your mind, at a later point in time, to easily refute your fears, frustrations and anxieties as they arise in your consciousness. Crayons and colored pencils may also stimulate your brain to create images, faces, doodles, and other self-expressions that reveal some important subconscious personal thought processes.

2. ***A quiet place, even a corner of a room, set aside to practice the exercises.***

Energy accumulates in a space that you set aside and use specifically for one purpose. Creating a special place for your own inner work is a strong suggestion to your subconscious, (the part of your brain that allows your dreams to germinate into fruition), that you are serious about transforming your life.

3. Recording Materials

Choose your own recording device.

To do the exercises in this book, you can read and stop, read and stop, or you can record your own voice first. Then you will be able to go straight through the exercise without stopping. The goal is for you to comfort yourself and love yourself. Hearing your own voice is a powerful affirmation that you can create what you want and you are all you will ever truly need.

As you begin your journey along the path to love, take a moment to assess where you are right now in your life. The questions you are about to answer may seem simple but are actually quite profound. Observe your thoughts. Notice any automatic body responses you may have. You are more than your thoughts. You are more than your body. Allow your automatic responses to help you to discover who you truly are.

For all the exercises in this introduction and in the rest of this book, you have choices. You can read the exercise and then write in your journal. You can record the entire exercise with your own voice, close the book, close your eyes, and visualize freely. Or, you can listen to the pre-recorded audio tapes that accompany each chapter.

Who Are You?

Sit in a comfortable position.

Inhale slowly, very slowly, and deeply.

Exhale slower than your usual rate.

Take three slow, deep, easy, and quiet breaths.

Close your eyes and allow your body to relax.

Take three more slow, deep, easy, and quiet breaths.

Open your eyes only to read each question.

Immediately close your eyes and allow the answer to come to you.

Accept the answers that come. Do not edit or change the response

Listen to your mind's first answer which is the most correct response at this moment.

Who am I?

What are other people here for in my life?

Why am I alive now?

What do I believe about love?

Who do I enjoy touching and for what purpose?

What yearns to heal inside of me?

What does sexual reawakening mean to me?

What is the role of God, a higher power, or spirituality in my life?

TABLE OF CONTENTS

PART TWO TOUCH *ME ... PLEASE*

TOUCH ME … PLEASE

BOOK TWO

INTRODUCTION

Touch me, please

I want to know you

Touch me … please

I don't know how

Touch me … please

We'll know each other

Touch me … please.

Your Body Believes You

Your body listens to every thought you have and every word you speak. And your body believes you. Your body speaks to you in body messages: sensations, pleasant and unpleasant, injuries, discomforts, aches and pains, and illnesses.

Other people recognize and respond to your body messages. You cannot hide who you are because every minute movement, expression and nuance is perceptible to anyone who sees you, regardless of whether they consciously know what they are seeing.

Whether you realize it or not, your five physical senses and your sixth intuitive sense are continually being stimulated by everyone and everything in your environment and beyond. You are literally touching and being touched by everyone and everything. The choice is actually very simple – to touch and be touched with conscious intention or unconsciously, with mindless lack of awareness.

Touch Me … Please, the second book in the ***Love Me, Touch Me, Heal Me*** Series, leads us on a path toward conscious, intentional touching … truly touching the heart and soul and spirit of everyone and everything, with all of our senses. Touch is the ultimate tool of intimacy, a no nonsense way of becoming close to another being. Touch is gentle, powerful, healing, all-knowing, deep, and reaches beyond any time, space or human concepts of boundaries. Touch allows us to overcome all obstacles and heal from whatever ails us. But the way most of us touch others and allow others to touch us, is often limited by our mental condition and personal beliefs. Touch is generous, magnanimous and offered freely to all who are receptive and in need. Touch is not for personal benefit, personal satisfaction, or personal gain. Touch is for interpersonal sharing, communication, intimate connection, love and healing.

Part Two is meant for people who touch, people who want to touch, people who want to be touched and people who want to touch again. You will have to explore your own bodily sensations, needs, cravings, desires and pleasures. You will also need to examine your personal thoughts, beliefs, attitudes, memories and dreams – to find the healing and loving touch, the most profoundly sensational touch, touch that you can bring into all aspects of your life. And you will be reminded, over and over, to bring that touch back to your own self so that you can fully share your healing and loving touch with your own self and with others.

****

TOUCH ME ... PLEASE

"The very strength that protects the heart from injury is the strength that prevents the heart from enlarging to its intended greatness within."

***The Treasured Writings of Kahlil Gibran*, Castle Books, P. 236**

Touch connects us to the world. Touch teaches. Touch heals. Sometimes touch hurts. Touch is powerfully intimate. Through touching and being touched, we feel. When we are touched with love, respect and gentle caring, our heart becomes open and receptive to love.

Through loving touch, we feel accepted, acknowledged, understood and loved. In Part II we look at our body and our senses, especially our sense of touch. We examine what we believe about touch, how we have touched and been touched, how we expect to be touched, and how we can create loving touch in our life. Here we are introduced to the various body therapies available that can help us to release whatever blocks us from the enjoyment of love, pleasure and health in our life.

TOUCH ME ... PLEASE

Touch Me ... Please

Touch me ...please
Reach inside
My mind
Turn the knob
To open the safe
Learn
The secret combination
To unleash
My inner truth

I will share myself
With you
Be patient
Be kind
Wait awhile
Discover
The subtle ways
I hide from you

We can be together
Right now
Giving love
Being love
Joyous
Happy
Let us
Open the door
To each other's hearts

Touch me
Feel my heart beat
See soft colors
Surrounding me
Love me
Love you
We are one
Our energies connect
We feel
We're alive
We're free

Touch me … please

TOUCH ME ... PLEASE

CHAPTER 1

YOUR BODY BELIEVES YOU

Your Body Believes You

Your body believes you

Tell it what you want it to hear

Your body speaks the truth

Listen to its wisdom

Your body is your temple

Honor it

Sanctify it

Love it

You and your body are one

Treat it as your beloved companion

It is yours for life.

Listen to Your Body

Your body listens to every thought you have, every word you speak. And your body believes you. Your body speaks to you in body messages: sensations, pleasant and unpleasant, injuries, discomforts, aches and pains, and illnesses.

Pay attention! Listen to the subtle messages your body offers you, moment to moment. Ignore these body messages (a knot in your stomach, a stubbed toe, an ache in your neck or shoulders) and the signals may intensify (full blown indigestion, a broken toe, whiplash, shoulder injury).

Your body sends us messages all the time. Physical symptoms are often a warning from your subconscious, reminding you to pay attention to your body or to some person, situation or life event.

- "Watch it! My heart is hurting from that person's remarks."
- "Look at that! I really can't stomach my work."
- "I have no support. My back is up against the wall."

Disease is not an external thing that happens to you. Disease is not a noun: "I **have** a cold, I **have** a cancer." Disease is a verb, an action, a happening, an allowing of something foreign to grow and develop, sometimes even with your own consent.

- “I am tensing my head, neck, back and allowing pain signals to intensify."
- “I am constricting my blood vessels, my nerves, my breathing."
- “I am straining my heart, my liver, my kidneys, my intestines."
- “I am supporting the growth of cancer cells in my body.”

Research with patients who display dissociative identity disorder, formerly called multiple personality disorder, have verified the power of our mind in our own illness. One personality could have all the symptoms of a disease, such as diabetes or skin rashes, while once another personality emerged, the doctors found absolutely no signs of that same illness, through blood tests and medical workups, in the very same person’s body. Disease is a messenger from your body/mind system. It is your body's attempt to heal itself by correcting imbalances and restoring harmony. A cold eliminates excess mucus. Almost like tears, it is your body's way of crying when life gets us down. A tumor or cyst is the body's attempt to encapsulate cells gone haywire.

When decoding the meaning behind a physical symptom in your body, always search for the physical causes first. Sometimes the cause is hereditary, genetic. Sometimes an injury is just that, an injury, or an infectious disease is just that, an infectious disease. After examining and exhausting the possible physical causes, then begin to look for possible emotional causes, beliefs and meanings in your own life. Examine your words, your verbal communication with and about your body.

Your body speaks your mind.

- Is something in your life eating away at you?
- Is something lying heavy in your gut?
- Are you unable to digest the meaning of an experience?

Use your words, your speech as a guide to your own unconscious. Pay attention to the words you use to describe you life and the sensations and symptoms in your body. Your underlying beliefs will become clear. And you may be amazed. Your words may match a symptom exactly. A highly regarded teacher of this unique Korean mind-body-spiritual method called Chun-Do-Sun-Bup, appeared one day using crutches. When I asked her how she had broken her leg, she replied: "I kept on saying, I lost my footing in America." Those were not just idle words. Her body actually responded to the way she was feeling.

Every thought and every emotion we have alters our immune system. Dr. Candace Pert, in her groundbreaking book, *Molecules of Emotion,* revealed that neurotransmitters travel fast throughout our body, into all of our body cells, not just in our brains, and are affected by our thoughts and emotions. It's not just the stressors in our life but how we interpret them and feel about them that creates our illnesses. Dr. Steven Locke of Harvard University Medical School found that natural killer cell activity is diminished, not by severe changes or stressors in healthy human volunteers, but by people's interpretations of the stress and whether they have a sense of being able to control or deal with it.

Your body speaks its mind. Illness often results from negative and ineffective communication between you and your body. Healing often happens when we develop effective conversation, a healing conversation. What are some of the conversations you have had with your own body recently, or on a regular basis?

- "He's making me sick." – stomachache
- "I can't stand it anymore." - leg or back problems
- "I wish I'd kept my big mouth shut" or "Nobody listens to me." - loss of voice
- "I can't listen to people's problems anymore" - hearing loss
- "I have to get out of here." - knee problems
- "I've lost my footing, my grounding" - broken foot or toe
- "Too many conflicting thoughts" - migraine headache

- "I can't take the steps I need to take in my life" - multiple schlerosis
- "That makes my blood boil." high blood pressure

Let Your Precious Body Speak To You

Sit quietly, in a comfortable position.

Place both of your feet securely on the ground.

Close your eyes and take an easy, slow, soft, deep breath.

Allow your mind to focus on your body.

Listen for those body signals that are loud and clear.

What do you notice first?

What part of your body is calling for your attention right now?

If more than one body part wants attention, **choose one part now.**

You may repeat this exercise again for other parts.

If this body part had a mind and a voice, what would it tell you about your life, your relationships, or your self?

Is something or someone causing you to feel pain, anger, frustration or some other upsetting emotion?

Sit quietly and breathe deeply.

If the answer is "No."

Appreciate any good feelings you may have.

Appreciate your body as your temple, your home.

If the answer is "Yes."

Ask yourself the following questions.

Allow the answers to come to you.

Just listen to the answers you receive without judging or censoring.

What has happened that you have allowed this person or situation to disturb you?

Is there something you've been trying that you've been unable to do?

What do you need to learn, change, practice, experience or study?

Imagine your body is your precious newborn baby.

Would you continually ignore your baby's cries for attention, food, or comfort?

Would you let your baby scream until he or she totally shut down?

Would you make your baby keep moving without any rest?

Would you deliberately deprive your baby of food and nourishment?

Listen to the message your body is sending you right now.

Stay quiet.

Reassure your body that you are indeed paying attention.

Imagine gently rocking and hugging your whole body.

Talk to Your Body

Talk to your body, either aloud or silently in your mind.

Ask your body what it wants and needs right now.

Talk to the parts that are injured, ill or hurting.

Discover what you can do to soothe yourself.

Talk to the parts that are old or no longer attractive.

Send them your unconditional love and acceptance.

Talk to your organs or body parts that are missing.

Send them your love, thank them for having served you in the past, and say goodbye to them now.

Talk to the tumors, cysts, cancers and other growths that have been removed.

Forgive them for any pain or problems they caused, thank them for what they have taught you, send them love, and say goodbye.

Talk to any unwanted cell growth on your body now.

Ask why the cells are growing and what lesson they might provide for you.

If you have had any miscarriages or abortions, talk to those unborn fetuses now.

Ask for their forgiveness, or say whatever you need to say, send them your love and say goodbye.

If your body has been abused, physically or sexually, by someone else, give your body the love, compassion, understanding and acceptance it has been craving.

If you have abused your body or have allowed it to be abused, physically or sexually, forgive yourself and give your body the caring love that it so desperately needs.

Is there anything else you want to tell your body now?

Promise to be kind to your body in thoughts and words and actions.'

Love Your Body

Love your body just the way it is.

Forgive your body for any changes, flaws, blemishes, weight changes, or other problems.

Love your body for its ability to adapt as it ages.

Love your body's size and shape.

Love the color and texture of your skin, hair and nails.

Love your fat, your scars, your freckles, your brown spots, your white spots, your purple scars and any other blatant damages.

Love all your organs, especially the troublesome ones.

Love all your organs or body parts that have been removed.

Love your wrinkles and frown lines that give your face expression.

Love your aches and pains for reminding you to pay attention.

Love your thinning hair, your bald spots, your saggy skin, pot belly, and cellulite.

Love your blemishes, burns, infections, and even rashes.

These are all reminders that you are alive, that your immune system is still working.

Once you have passed on, your body will no longer feel pain, there will be no more wrinkles, blemishes and other growths. There will no longer be a body.

Love your body

Love your body

Love your body

It is the only one you have

Your body is the temple for your soul

Love it

Honor it

Appreciate it

Be amazed by its intricate detail and magnificent coordination

Allow your body to heal

IN A MOMENT YOU WILL BE ASKED TO TOUCH YOUR BODY.

This simple gesture can have a profound and lasting effect. For some of you this may be a new, and even scary, experience. Honor yourself. Don't push. If anything you're asked to do doesn't feel right or safe for you, STOP THE EXERCISE IMMEDIATELY! Put a sticker on this page, reminding your self to return to this exercise at some future time.

Touch and Soothe Your Precious Body

Imagine your body is your precious newborn baby.

Send the following loving thoughts to your body.

"I love you. I will soothe and take care of you from now on."

Allow one hand to gently touch and soothe your body, part by part.

Now let your other hand gently glide all over your body.

Notice which body parts you touch, don't touch or tentatively touch.

Notice any differences in sensation, feelings and thoughts when your body is touched by your right hand or your left hand.

Gently rub and soothe and rock your body, thinking how much you love it.

Notice how your body feels right now.

Your body reveals to you the mystery of life. Your body warns you of impending danger through fear, pain and automatic fight or flight responses. Your body impels you to connect with other humans through our thoughts, hearts and hands. Most of us search endlessly for pleasurable sensations, love and physical contact. Some of us have learned to fear pleasure, deny love, and avoid human contact. Within every cell, our body retains memories of all the sensations, thoughts and emotions we have experienced in this lifetime and perhaps even before.

At times we treat our body as if it is not part of us. For a moment of pleasure or purposely to dull our conflicted and stressed out mind, we may eat, drink, inhale or inject substances that over-stimulate, suppress, or clog up our bodily systems. We often push our self to keep going when our body is begging for rest. We ignore our aching muscles and continue working or playing sports until injury strikes. Most of us would never consider putting the wrong type of gasoline in our automobile or an inferior brand of detergent in our washing machine. Why then, do we so often neglect to give our own body the food, rest and love that we know will enhance our health?

Health is no longer a mystery. We now know a lot about attaining and maintaining good health. Containing all of our organs, our body represents us to the world. How we love and nurture our body determines who we ultimately become.

Food Is The Fuel of Life

Food is the fuel of life. Without adequate nutrients, our mind is unfocused, we become fidgety, irritable, and tired. Without good enough nutrition, we are not able to function at an optimal level. It's that simple. It is well-documented that we need carbohydrates for quick energy, fat for more sustained energy, protein to build and repair tissues, vitamins, minerals, trace elements and water to maintain a healthy immune system.

Knowing the essential value of food, why do we often choose to not nourish our body? Why do we crave unhealthy foods and over-indulge in foods that may otherwise be good for us? Why are so many of us addicted to drugs, cigarettes, alcohol, caffeine or sugar? We know the dangers of continuing our habits: depleting our vitamins and minerals, decreasing our breathing capacity, interfering with our brain functioning, and lowering our immune system. What is it that prevents many of us from choosing an optimal balance of healthy foods to sustain our body?

Your Favorite Food

Open to a new page in your journal and write the words at the top: My Favorite Foods.

List your 10 favorite foods.

What is it about these foods that you like (color, taste, texture, fragrance, memories evoked, or the way you feel during or after eating)?

What emotions do you feel before, while eating, and after eating your favorite foods?

List your 10 least favorite foods.

What is it about these foods that you dislike (color, taste, texture, fragrance, memories evoked, or the way you feel during or after eating)?

What emotions do you feel before, while eating, and after eating your least favorite foods?

Eating Your Favorite Food

Imagine one of your favorite foods.

Visualize the color, texture, appearance, shape, and fragrance.

Imagine taking a bite. Savor the taste as it passes your lips and tongue and travels down your esophagus toward your stomach.

Notice how your body feels as you soak in the fragrance and taste and feel the

texture of this delicious food.

Inside Your Favorite Food

Imagine this favorite food is growing larger right before your eyes.

Take a fantasy trip right into the center of this favorite food.

Imagine this food surrounding all of your cells.

Feel the sensation of your body being enveloped by this food.

Describe your thoughts, feelings and sensations?

For example, "You soothe me when I feel anxious."

"You comfort me when I'm upset."

"You're with me when I feel lonely."

Imagine stepping outside of this food into a warm, clean shower.

Allow your body to feel clean and tingly all over.

Drawing Your Favorite Food

On a clean sheet of paper or in your journal, draw a picture of your favorite food.

Now draw yourself near this food, eating or playing with it, resisting it, ignoring it, squashing it or climbing inside of it.

Describe your thoughts, sensations, and reactions to this food now.

Food as Your Best Friend

Imagine that this food is your best friend, your lover, or a very close relative.

Have a conversation.

Talk to this food about your attraction to it and the benefits of your friendship.

Find out if there are any problems between you. Have a real intimate discussion. For example, "You're always here when I need a friend." "You help me forget or ignore my problems when I'm upset."

This food may be jealous and keep you away from other food that is good for you.

Talk to this food about your fears.

"Sometimes I'm afraid you control me."

"You have the power to fill me up and prevent me from eating other foods that I need to maintain my health."

"If I eat too much of you, I may gain weight, become lethargic, lose my appetite for other foods."

What have you discovered about your relationship to food?

What have you learned about your relationship to your favorite foods and your least favorite foods?

Food has a profound effect upon your life. Some of us live for our next meal, preparing, talking, even dreaming about the taste and sensual pleasure of eating. Years ago, I spent Christmas week with a boyfriend and his family. From a traditional ethnic background, his family sat around the table talking about food for hours and hours. His overweight mother complained about her difficulty keeping a diet. She spent most of her days shopping, cooking, tasting, talking about, and serving food. How could she possibly lose weight without changing her lifestyle and affecting the comfort of her family?

On the other hand, there are others of us who are overly disciplined about our eating. We carefully select only the most essential foods. Limiting our portions, we eat bland and raw foods, vegetable juices, fiber drinks, whole grains, abundant fruits and vegetables, and very limited desserts, sugar, oils or salt. Being cautious about our eating, we make sure to eat slowly, chew our food carefully, stop eating before we are completely full, plan our meal schedules and prepare foods to take with us during the day. We may be physically healthy. We may live longer lives than the more sensual eaters. But, perhaps, we are denying ourselves one of the truly great pleasures of life, **Food**.

Recent studies have found that people who ate dessert once or twice a week were actually healthier than those who never ate dessert. In a stress management class, I asked my students to list their favorite foods. Nobody listed broccoli, bean sprouts, or tofu. The students' favorite foods were chocolate cake, ice cream, pizza, cheese, spaghetti, and mashed potatoes. Their favorite foods were emotionally soothing and pleasing to the taste buds.

Denying yourself the pleasure of food may symbolize the way you live your life. If you deny yourself food, you may also tend to limit your emotional involvement, deny your deepest emotions, and ignore your body's messages.

For some of us, some of the time, food is our only friend, our solace in times of need. Food can look good, smell good, taste good, calm our emotions, and comfort us. For others, food can be our way of hurting our self, damaging our body, proving how tough we are, or gaining control over something. In extreme cases, such as anorexia nervosa and bulemia, our relationship to food can take over our life, interfere with intimacy, and threaten our very existence. For others, chemical substances such as alcohol, recreational drugs, and prescription drugs can become our favorite food, interfering with the health of our mind, body and spirit.

Exercise Moves Your Life

Some of us fill our body with the most powerful and healing nutrients. At the same time, we may either avoid exercise or overtax our muscles through excessive exercise, improper body alignment, or not enough stretching to keep us limber. Some of us are afraid to exercise, afraid of the pain, discomfort, and normal sweating. Some of us exercise moderately, eat a healthy, balanced diet, yet we may still manage to injure our body through repetitive patterns of overuse.

As far back as I can remember, I was always athletic, climbing trees and hiking in the woods, skating, skiing, dancing, and playing team sports. Although physical activity was pleasurable, even exciting to me, I thought being athletic and physically fit meant pain, perpetual pain. I had a tendency to overdo a good thing, not knowing when to stop.

How Do You Exercise Your Body?

What are your favorite physical activities?

Do you enjoy working out and exercising your body?

What influenced you to enjoy or not enjoy exercising your body?

How do you usually feel when you exercise regularly?

How do you usually feel when you don't exercise regularly?

Our body not only belongs to us, it **is** us. Without our body, we would no longer exist as the person we know our self to be. Some of us attempt to live separately from our own body, as if that were possible. We continually ignore our body's messages. We refuse to accept our God-given shape, health, fitness or advancing age.

Observing Your Body

Get ready to look at your body.

Remember to use soft and gentle eyes.

Your goal is to observe and evaluate - not to judge and criticize.

Stand in front of a full length mirror.

You can choose to observe yourself fully dressed, partially clothed or totally undressed.

Have a conversation with yourself looking back at you in the mirror.

Describe what you see.

Talk as if you were telling your own little child how he or she looks.

Speak to the person in the mirror as gently and kindly as you can.

What do you find is attractive, appealing, sexy, youthful, charming...?

What do you find is unattractive, fat, skinny, soft, hard, unappealing...."

Tell the person in the mirror what you like best and least about your body.

Imagine your body parts responding to your words.

What do you body parts want to tell you?

Notice how you feel as you observe and talk about your own body.

Listen to your body's subtle and not so subtle responses.

Inside Your Body

Imagine for a moment your consciousness could travel into the center of your body.

How do you feel inside your body?

Do you feel restricted, compressed, shocked, over-stimulated, exhausted, or depressed?

Do you feel happy, free, joyful, elated, or ecstatic?

Now, imagine travelling inside your own body.

Explore your organs (liver, kidneys, bladder, pancreas, spleen, heart, lungs, small intestine, large intestine, urinary tract, reproductive organs [uterus, testes], external sexual organs [penis, vagina], anal canal). Explore your nervous system (brain, spinal cord, cerebrospinal fluid, membranes, spinal nerves emanating toward your organs, nerve plexuses).

Explore the muscles, tendons, ligaments and bones throughout your body, from your head, scalp, face, neck, shoulders, arms, hands, fingers and upper torso to your lower body, legs, feet and toes.

Explore the liquids (blood, lymph, water, and cerebrospinal fluid) flowing through your arteries, veins and interstitial spaces.

In what places do you get stuck and find you cannot move?

In what places do you move easily and effortlessly?

In what places do you move too easily, without enough boundary or separation?

Which parts do you pay most attention to?

Which parts do you ignore?

Which parts are you afraid of, ashamed of, proud of, neutral about, or angry at?

What would it take for you to become intimate with every part of your own body?

What Do You Want To Change About Your Body?

Tell yourself in the mirror what you would like to change about your body.

Don't worry right now about how you will accomplish this change.

Don't think about whether or not you believe the change is possible.

Just tell the truth about what you would like to change.

Talk to yourself about current activites that affect your weight, fitness, health and body image.

What are you currently doing that you wish to continue?

What activities, habits would you like to stop doing?

What activities, habits would you like to add to your life?

Body Image Analysis Chart

In your journal, create the following chart and put a check mark in the appropriate column for each body part.

	Love It	**Not Happy But Can't Change**	**Want To Change**
Attractiveness			
Face			
Hair			
Eyes			
Mouth			
Chin			
Ears			
Neck			
Shoulders			
Arms			
Chest			
Back			
Waist			
Abdomen			
Hips			
Buttocks			
Thighs			
Calves			
Ankles			

Feet

Toes

Posture

Other

Describe Your Body

In your journal, answer the following questions about your body.

What do I like about my body?

What are the most attractive parts of my body?

What are the least attractive parts of my body?

What body parts am I most proud of?

What body parts am I ashamed of?

What are my strongest body parts?

What are my weakest body parts?

What is the most vulnerable, most easily injured, part of my body?

What body parts have been injured, broken, operated upon?

Where do I habitually carry tensions in my body?

In what areas of my body am I most flexible?

In what areas of my body am I least flexible?

What habitual thoughts and actions enhance my body image?

What habitual thoughts and actions destroy my body image?

What would I like to change about my body?

What do I believe I would have to do to make that change happen?

What could I do now to become more satisfied with my body image?

Your Body Outline

Draw a large outline of your body. If possible, lie down on a life size sheet of paper and have a friend or partner draw your an actual outline of your body.

With colored pencils or crayons, express the emotions of each body part. Write the words or an image that each body part would say or express if it had a voice.

Now, in your journal, answer the following questions about your body.

How do you habitually hold and carry your body?

What purpose does each part of your body have for you in your life?

Do your tense back muscles help you keep up a good front while your back is up against the wall?

Do your shoulders allow you to carry on by holding onto problems?

Do you dig your toes into the ground to hold your position?

What thoughts, emotions, sensations do you regularly feel?

What thoughts, emotions, sensations do you avoid feeling?

When was the last time you:

- *laughed a hysterical belly laugh?*
- *threw a temper tantrum, screamed and jumped up and down?*
- *punched a person or banged a pillow in raging anger?*
- *giggled in mischievous delight?*
- *cried at a sad movie?*
- *told someone your deepest fears, your secret longings, your private pleasures?*
- *allowed yourself to follow your own dream?*

Your body is your teacher. Pay attention to its messages. Explore the hidden meanings. Take a peak inside yourself. Discover what you truly feel and who you really are.

Caring For Your Body

Our body is a finely tuned machine. The parts can work throughout our entire life. However, in the same way that a machine requires proper care, oiling, checkups, part replacements, and to not be overused or abused, our body also requires adequate care throughout our life.

Each of our body systems needs to be maintained. Although no one bodily system is more important than any other, our breathing apparatus and how we use it can create or solve many of our health problems. Proper breathing allows our blood to circulate freely bringing nutrients to all of our cells. Breathing allows our central nervous system to signal our muscles to move and our pituitary gland to regulate our hormones. Breathing allows our autonomic nervous system to stimulate our vital organs to circulate blood, take in oxygen and eliminate stale air, digest, store, receive nutrients from our food, and eliminate toxins and waste products. Breathing allows our body to become sexually aroused, to build to a crescendo of passion, and to have a release of sexual energy that spreads peace, calm and relaxation throughout our bodily cells. Breathing allows us to feel our loving and tender emotions, synchronize our bodily rhythms, and connect intimately with our partner.

Many of us have long ago forgotten how to breathe. Just watch a baby breathe the "happy baby breath," a term coined by leading breath work expert, Gay Hendricks. A baby's head moves back and its belly rises up as it arches into a full abdominal breath and releases into a relaxed wide open back. Normal, healthy babies do not restrict their breathing. Abused, traumatized and neglected babies reflexively contract, constrict and become despondent. Restricted breathing is one of the major deterrents to a flexible body, peaceful mind, and loving, pleasurable sexuality.

Breath Is Life

Life begins when we take our first breath and ends when we breathe for the last time. We can live for weeks without food or sleep and days without water. Unless we are advanced yogis who can retain their breath for 1/2 hour or longer, if we are deprived of oxygen for only a few minutes, we will die. Deep and rhythmical breathing nourishes our body cells, assisting fluids and basic nutrients to be absorbed into our tissues and organs. When we restrict our breathing, our cells do not fully receive nourishment. Our body becomes inflexible, our muscles tense, our posturing armored, and we find our self agitated, easily frightened, even panicked.

If your breathing is full and you spot danger, your heart rate quickens and your breathing becomes more shallow. You inhale and exhale in a shorter range. When the danger passes, your breathing soon returns to normal. If your breathing is already restricted, the slightest perceived danger can prompt a panic reaction. Panic (intense anxiety and shortness of breath) often results when shallow, restricted breathing is restricted a bit more. Your brain may interpret the restricted breathing as severe danger, even dying. As human beings we are equipped to breathe deeply when we want to relax, to conserve our breathing when we are under attack or in a state of danger, to retain our breath for a length of time, to breathe through each of our nostrils instead of mainly through our mouth, and to regulate and vary our breathing as the situation requires. Flexibility and variability in our breathing mirrors the flexibility and variability in our life. Changing the way we breathe affects our thoughts and our emotions. Changing the way we breathe transforms our life.

Observing Your Breathing

Observe yourself breathing.

Begin by sitting comfortably in a chair with your feet placed firmly on the ground.

Listen for the sounds of your inhale and exhale.

Describe the quality of your breath (deep and full, short and shallow).

Are you actually holding your breath, resisting breathing?

Which is longer and fuller, your inhale or your exhale?

Are you breathing through your mouth, your nose, one or both nostrils?

Is your breathing quiet or forceful, smooth or choppy, loud or soft?

Is there any pain, tension or discomfort as you breathe?

What parts of your body move as you sit and breathe?

Which parts of your body are touching or not touching the chair as you breathe?

Now find a comfortable place to lie flat on your back, preferably on a cushion, mat, a couch or a bed.

Listen for the sounds of your inhale and exhale.

Describe the quality of your breath (deep and full, short and shallow).

How is your breathing the same or different now that you are lying on your back?

What parts of your body move as you lie flat on your back and breathe?

Is there any pain, tension or discomfort as you breathe?

Which parts of your body are touching or not touching the floor or mat as you breathe?

Now come to a comfortable standing position with your feet facing forward, about shoulder width apart, your knees ever so slightly bent.

Feel the soles of your feet spreading out, every part contacting the ground.

Bring your awareness to your each of your toes, the inside arch, the balls of your feet, your heels, and your ankles.

Listen for the sounds of your inhale and exhale.

Describe the quality of your breath (deep and full, short and shallow).

How is your breathing the same or different now that you are standing?

What parts of your body move as you stand and breathe?

Is there any pain, tension or discomfort as you breathe?

Which parts of your feet are touching the floor where you are standing?

Now begin to move your body.

Notice how your breathing shifts and changes as you move.

Bend, reach, stretch, twist and turn.

Walk, run, hop, skip, and jump.

Put on some music and let your body dance.

In your journal, describe what happens to your breathing as you move your body in different ways.

Most of us are unaware of our habitual breathing patterns. Many of us allow our shoulders to slump forward, constricting and compressing our ribs, chest and lung capacity. In this position, we can hardly take in enough air, inhaling and exhaling quickly but not deeply, in order to survive. Some of us have been taught to "stand up straight." So, we proudly lift and expand our chest, constricting our back muscles and ribs. In this position, we may be able to inhale deeply, but we cannot fully exhale. We can literally become stuck in our own breath. Some of us breathe up into our clavicles and chest, our abdomens tightening in the process. This type of breathing can keep us in a perpetual state of readiness to fight, to run, and to spot any danger in our environment. Some of us are perpetual deep abdominal breathers, so relaxed that we fail to garner up the required energy for a hard day's work.

The way we breathe has a powerful effect upon the way we live our life. Constricted breathing reflects fear and insecurity in our thoughts and emotions. Full, deep, regulated breathing reflects control, confidence and joy in our everyday life.

We can control our thoughts and feelings by changing the way we breathe. We can also control our breathing, by changing our thoughts.

Minding Your Body

Our mind controls our body and affects all the events of our life. It is not what actually happens to us that ultimately counts, but how we perceive what happens and how we recall it later. Our body is continually bombarded with incoming stimulation. All sensory input is recorded in our cells. Our mind selectively interprets, judges, and evaluates the encoded data. We cannot possibly remember and focus on all incoming sensations. But, long after the stimulation has been withdrawn and our conscious mind has forgotten the experience, our body retains the memory.

If the circuits in our brain are functioning properly, we will automatically perceive incoming stimulation accurately. We will recognize pain, pleasure, and other stimuli, and respond appropriately. For some of us, however, as we grew up, pleasurable and painful sensations were at times intermingled with abandonment, rejection, sexual abuse, and even, love. Our mind may have become confused. It's as if our circuits have crossed and our brain signals are scrambled. We may have lost our ability to interpret incoming stimulation accurately. We may actually perceive pleasure as pain, love as abuse, or touch as rejection. Losing the brain connection to our body, we may actually behave as if our body is separate from our mind and thoughts.

If the stimulation we received was intense or overwhelming to us, we may have learned to block our ability to interpret or even feel certain sensations. Our body may feel numb in response to pain or pleasure. Wilhelm Reich, colleague of Freud and forerunner of body psychotherapy, coined the term "body armoring" to describe this phenomenon. Resulting from specific stimuli, life events, and our personal responses and interpretations, most of us develop a habitual way of holding our body. Depending upon where in our body we have developed armoring, different emotions and thought processes may be blocked from our conscious awareness.

Armoring yourself does not prevent stimulation from reaching your senses. It merely blocks your mind's ability to recognize and respond appropriately. Armoring allows you to maintain the semblance of a healthy, organized existence. However, one intense life event, touching or being touched, sexual arousal, falling in love, abusing or being abused, feeling rejected, returning home from war, or even giving birth to a child, can temporarily shatter your armoring. Emotions you didn't even know you had can come crashing to the surface, literally causing you to have an emotional breakdown.

Many of us will do almost anything to avoid facing our hidden feelings and the possibility of breaking down. Chemical and sexual addictions are the most obvious. But some of the most positive and constructive activities: career building, exercise, shopping, travelling, even reading, can also be used to numb our mind and prevent us from facing our feelings.

No amount of stimulation and activity can help us to avoid our deepest feelings for our entire life - for decades perhaps, but not forever. Lying in a hospital bed with less than three weeks to live, my mother finally faced the feelings she had avoided and dreaded all of her life. When she could no longer escape into activity, she finally confronted her self, her fears, and her life. She cried every day. Terrified of dying, she was afraid to feel the fear and pain she had never allowed herself to embrace in her 76 years of living. It wasn't until her final day on earth that she came to terms with her own life. Reaching a point of acceptance, she finally said, "I feel encouraged."

You and I do not have to wait until we have only a few weeks left to live. We have the opportunity to assess and review our life, right now, and at regular intervals, while we are fully alive and fully active. We can begin by observing our thoughts, discriminating between what is true for us and what is merely repetition of other people's beliefs.

How do we ultimately discover our own truth? The answer is very simple. Our emotions do not lie. Without premeditated effort, when we feel wronged, we get angry. When we feel hurt or rejected, we become sad. When we feel excited and stimulated, we feel happy. Sometimes our thoughts tell us not to listen to our emotions. Perhaps we have learned that it is not okay to smile and feel pleasure; it is better to be serious. Perhaps we have learned not to express anger; it is better to remain calm, cool, and accepting. Perhaps we have learned not to allow our self to feel sad; it is better to put on a happy, contented expression or to keep a stiff upper lip as we quietly endure the inevitable suffering. Listen to your emotions. They will provide answers that cannot be obtained from any other source.

Your Emotions Are Your Best Friends

Your emotions are your best friends. They arrive at just the right moment. Pay attention. Your emotions are messengers from your higher self. Listen and they may remind you about something you have been ignoring, avoiding, or refusing to see in your life. Pleasant emotions may tell you that you are okay right now, you are on the right path. Painful or debilitating emotions may force you to halt your current activity, disconnect from friends, acquaintances, and lovers, or prepare to leave your current job.

Neurobiologists have isolated some of the brain functions responsible for imprinting a traumatic event in the subconscious while blocking that event from the conscious mind. Studies show that intense emotions interfere with our ability to process information and behave appropriately.

Quantum physicists describe our emotions as energy particles. If not released through expression, these particles can become trapped in our body, in the spaces between the atoms. Sexual and physical abuse, trauma, and intense emotions may cause us to naturally constrict our breathing and tense our muscles. When the excitation becomes overwhelming, our brain may not be able to process the information accurately. The trauma may remain embedded in our physical body, while the emotions become dull and blocked. When our brain circuits are overloaded, we may experience temporary amnesia, inability to remember our experiences. As adults, we may recall, in detail, the events of a traumatic episode, an emotional upset, or even physical abuse, but we may find our self unable to feel any emotions about the memory. Erroneously, we may believe that we were not emotionally affected. In reality, intense emotions may be lying dormant in our subconscious, waiting for the proper moment to explode outward.

It takes a certain amount of life energy to encapsulate our emotions and keep them hidden from our conscious mind. Our body is a hologram. Every part affects every other part. When any part is constricted, other muscles, organs and our entire nervous system must work overtime to maintain the homeostasis of our living and functioning body.

Your Life Force

You have a body and a mind. Your breathing keeps you alive. Food sustains you. Exercise energizes and strengthens you. Your mind controls you. But there is something more, some unseen force that enables you to thrive and flourish or to struggle and suffer. This life force, energy or spirit, has been recognized by most cultures. The Yogis call it "kundalini,"

Sigmund Freud called it "life instinct," Wilhelm Reich labeled it "orgone energy." A rose by any other name still smells the same. Whatever it is called, it is one and the same energy, and all of us have it. In many of us, this powerful force lies dormant, waiting to be awakened. For others, it has been awakened, yet we continually attempt to control, suppress or ignore it. And for the lucky few, this life force energy is harnessed, savored, and used to create whatever is most desired in life: love, professional recognition, financial comfort, family, emotional well-being, and sexual intimacy.

Where Is Your Life Force?

Sit quietly and close your eyes. Breathe slowly, deeply and effortlessly.

Locate your life force.

Scan through your body.

Where do you most strongly feel your life force, the energy that sustains you and propels you into action?

Now, consciously move your life force.

Allow your life force to travel downward towards your feet and toes.

Become aware of your feet and your entire body connecting with the grounding earth.

Feel the earth's magnetic power spreading through the muscles, tissues and reflexes in the soles of your feet.

Allow your life force to begin to move upwards through your legs, pelvic area, torso, and into your arms and shoulders.

Raise your arms above your head, allowing your life force to move upwards toward your hands and fingers.

Now, allow your life force to radiate outward from the top of your head and the tips of your fingers toward the energy of the sun, the moon, the planets, the stars, and the entire universe.

Now, gathering strength from celestial energy, allow your life force to re-enter your body from above, through the top of your head and the tips of your fingers.

Pull your life force down into your neck and shoulders, torso and center of your body.

Now, allow your life force to emanate outward from the center of your body, your hara, your belly, the container for most of your vital organs.

Feel the strength and power of your own life force to enter and return from the world outside.

Now raise your life force up to your heart as your feel your heart beat with your own life force.

Now, allow your life force to emanate outward from your heart. Feel the joy and wonder and ecstasy of connecting your heart to all the energies around you - people, plants, animals, and non-living, manmade forms of all sorts. Bring your life force back into your body. Allow the energy to spread through all your cells. Feel your cells opening, smiling, even laughing at the joy and wonder of you.

Retain your life force inside your body. Feel your own power and connection to the source, to life, and to everything that is.

We are more than our physical body. Every cell contains our spirit. Our body is the container for our soul. Why not allow our soul to love and touch us now? We will never *need* anyone else again. Of course, we may prefer to share our life, our body and our sensual pleasures with another person, but we will not *need* them to make us feel good. Let's love our self now. Honor our self. We will then know with total certainty that we are loved, that we can be touched and held any time we choose, that we can heal from whatever ails us, and that we are not alone.

Loving Yourself

Stand or sit in front of a mirror.

Tell yourself the words you are longing to hear from someone who loves you.

Say to yourself,

"I love you, my precious angel, sweet darling dearest jewel."

"I love you, powerful leader, intelligent dreamer, exquisite lover."

Tell yourself all those poetic, dramatic, loving, romantic words and phrases from your favorite Hollywood movies.

Tell yourself the loving, respectful, joyful words you may believe are only meant

for others who are more beautiful, more creative, more wealthy, more connected, more clever, more cultured, more powerful, or more deserving than you.

Repeat to yourself those loving words that someone told you, long ago.

Tell yourself all those words you've never heard before.

Gaze into your own eyes in the mirror.

Take five or ten long, slow, deep, rhythmical breaths.

Breathe in the feeling and power of these tender, loving words meant only for you.

Love and Touch Your Body

Continue to breathe slowly and deeply at a steady pace.

Gaze into your own eyes in the mirror.

Begin to touch and caress your body, part by part, all over your body surface.

If your touch becomes sensual or even sexual, allow that to happen naturally.

Keep repeating loving words to your own image in the mirror.

"I love you my dearest darling, precious angel."

"You are the salt of the earth, the god or goddess of the heavens, the entrance to the river of love."

"You are beautiful and radiant."

"Your soul shines brightly."

"You are the dream of every man and the heart's desire of every woman."

"You are the flame of my life."

"You are the one true love I have been searching for, waiting for all my life."

"You are with me now and I will never leave you."

If you find it difficult to create your own romantic words, read aloud the words above or words from your favorite poems, novels, plays or movies. Buy a book of love poems. Pablo Neruda's, Kahlil Gibran's, and Rumi's love poems are exquisite.

Read the poems aloud as you gaze into the wondrous, beautiful eyes in this mirror of

your own life.

Tell the person in the mirror how much in love you are and that you will remain in love forever.

Always be there for yourself

Love yourself.

Honor yourself.

Breathe your body.

Touch your body.

Clear your mind.

Awaken your spirit.

Listen to your heart.

Your body believes you

Tell it what you want it to hear

Always be there for yourself

And you will wake up singing

The sweetest and most powerful

Poignant melody of life

Your life

Right here

Right now

IT'S A

SENSATIONAL WORLD

TOUCH ME … PLEASE

CHAPTER 2

IT'S A SENSATIONAL WORLD

It's A Sensational World

My tongue has tasted
Better days
My throat collapsed
From closed up ways
Half opened eyes
Refuse to see
This beautiful world
Especially me

I hear the sounds
Of laughter calling
On the ground
My knees are crawling
Shoulders ache
My neck is tight
My poor back spasms
I shake with fright

All because
My body tells me
Everything
I need to know
Full sensation
Living, breathing
Listen to me
Let me go

Lift my shoulders
To the heavens
Open up
My hungry throat
Let me speak
From deep within me
Hear the wisdom
Of my soul

My mind pretends
To have the answers
My mind believes
It has to know
Let my mind
Release its thinking
Let my thoughts
Begin to slow

Life surrounds me
Joy and sorrow
Filling up
My soulful heart
Crying, laughing
Sad, now angry
Raw emotions
Stop and start

Touch my heart
With joy and wonder
Let me know
I'll be okay
I will feel
All life's sensations
Knowing
I'm alive today.

Living Is Feeling

It's a sensational world! Living is feeling. We feel the beauty and wonder of this world with all of our senses. Being fully alive is feeling pleasure and feeling pain, allowing our self to explore the heights of joy and also delve into the depths of darkness, the parts of our self and others that we wish did not exist. Often it is precisely these deep dark painful feelings and emotions that catapult our creative urges to fruition. If we seek to dampen and dull our painful feelings, we are in danger of also limiting our joie de vivre, our creative spirit, our compassion, our sensitivity, and our passionate enjoyment of life.

Imagine animals in the wild or our beloved pets in our homes, taking drugs to suppress their fears, to boost their energy, or to allow their bodies to relax. Cats and dogs, fish and birds, horses, rabbits, elephants, and all animals do not need drugs to accept themselves. They do not avoid feeling their emotions. Tigers and fawns, lions and kangaroos, insects and mice, and all animals utilize their feelings, both positive and negative, for their very survival. They use their hostile and aggressive feelings to obtain food, fight off attackers, and to protect their territory and the weaker members of their species. They use their fearful emotions to guide them to seek safety for themselves and their young ones. Their positive feelings lead them to play in their natural environment while their bodies secrete pheromones to attract mates, ensuring the survival of their species.

Observe animals moving their bodies through space, frolicking in the natural sensations of life. Watch a carefree bird gracefully and effortlessly flap its wings as it soars across the open sky. See another bird peacefully float atop the waves on a windy sea, allowing the water to splash upon its feathers, obviously enjoying the experience.

Watch a happy dog go charging, over and over and over again, to retrieve an object tossed by its human companion. See an excitedly barking dog run to greet its caretaker, jumping up to lick it's owner's face, wagging its tail rapidly back and forth, its body expressing total joy in the moment. Feel the softness of a loving cat's fur as it rubs up against your leg. Listen to the soothing sound of the cat purring contentedly as you lift it to rest in your lap.

It's a Sensational World

Join me now on a sensual fantasy into your own mind and body. Imagine yourself being carefree as a wild animal, contentedly enjoying your surroundings and all the sensations of life. Close your eyes. Take a few slow, deep, and full breaths. Allow your body to relax and your mind to be open to new possibilities. Now, imagine you are peacefully lying outdoors on a full-length lounge chair. Feel the warmth of the sun heating up your sunscreen oiled skin. Sense your muscles relax as your thoughts drift away and your mind becomes more and more still. Now, imagine you are walking on a hot sandy beach, tip toeing quickly to avoid burning the bottoms of your sensitive feet. In front of you is a body of cool water. Quickly dip your toes in, feeling a rush of cold tingle along your legs, sending a shiver up your spine. As you slowly sink your whole body down into the cool water, feel the goose bumps in your skin as your body begins to shake. Rapidly move your arms and legs and feel your own blood rushing through your vessels as your body begins to warm up. Soon you emerge from the water, refreshed and exuberant.

Walk back in the sand, forming deep footprints as you walk, the soles of your feet firmly planted with each step. Climb down into a nearby jacuzzi. Feel your aches and pains soak away in the heated fragrant bubbling jet streams. Hold onto a cool glass of ice water as you plunk an ice cube into your mouth. Suck on the ice cube and allow the coolness to numb your tongue and lips and inner cheeks. Take a sip of the water and feel the cooling sensation of fluid flowing down the center of your dry, parched throat. Climb out of the hot tub and enter a steaming hot shower. Feel the prickling goodness of the clean hot water as you lather up your body, part by part, massaging your scalp and hair with fragrant herbal soap. Step into soft cushion slippers as you rub your body briskly with an oversize terry cloth towel.

Slip your body into a comfortable outfit of natural soft cotton clothing. Return to your room and open the wrapper of a small piece of exquisite chocolate. Taste the soothing texture and flavor as the chocolate slowly melts in your mouth. Now, quickly pack your bags, call a taxi, and head for the airport. Listen to the cacophony of sounds as your taxi glides through the traffic and the weather changes to a gentle rain. Listen to the horns blasting, sirens screeching, people yelling, motors running, and cars skidding.

Look at your watch and discover you are running late and may even miss your flight. Notice how your heart is racing and your body is becoming tense. Finally, you arrive at the airport, pay the driver, grab your bags, and go through the baggage check line. Observe your own impatience as you are asked to open your bag while others breeze through undisturbed. Stand on the side, rearrange the contents of your suitcase, close the bag, pull up the handle and roll away as you race walk toward your gate. Breathless and excited, feel a relieved smile spread across your face as you hand your boarding pass to the gate attendant. Board the plane, twisting and turning as you maneuver your body and bag down the narrow aisle until you find your seat. Place your bag in the overhead bin, sit down, buckle your seat belt, and wait in quiet anticipation. Listen to the roaring sound of the engine as the plane taxis down the runway. Now the plane is positioned for takeoff. Sit back and breathe deeply as you watch the nose of the plane begin to rise.

Sensation Is The Language Of The Body

This is your life! How do you want to live it? Sensation is the language of the body, reminding us in every moment that we have a body and that our body is alive and breathing and filled with sensation. We live in a world of continual sensation. One of the cruelest forms of punishment is to keep a person isolated, in a dark narrow space, with no room to move about, devoid of light, sound, and other sensual stimulation. In such a state of sensual deprivation, our mind and thought processes will rapidly deteriorate. Children who do not receive adequate stimulation do not thrive. They become depressed, despondent, and eventually die. Studies conducted at The Crêche, a home for orphans in Lebanon in the 1950's, revealed that receiving only minimal amounts of stimulation, the infants, called foundlings, laid in bed without the usual energy and interest in the world that most children display. Their intellectual development was severely stunted and they remained mentally retarded for life. However, those foundlings who were adopted before the age of two years old, regained their full mental capacity for the rest of their lives.

To survive and thrive and develop satisfying productive lives, we require daily stimulation of all of our senses. Internally, we are aware of our need to cough, sneeze, hiccup, scratch an itch, resist being tickled, belch or relieve gas. We feel and even hear our stomach gurgle when we are hungry or when our body is in the process of digesting food we have already eaten. We feel goose bumps cover our body when we are frightened, startled, or have made an important discovery or realization. We are often aware of tension or pain in our body, although we do not always know the exact origin.

Sometimes we are conscious of the way we are breathing. We may notice that we are breathing rapidly, holding our breath in fear or anxiety, gasping in horror and disbelief, or breathing a sigh of relief about some important situation. We are also aware of our emotions as they well up inside of us, forcing a response such as laughter, tears, disappointment, anger, or even rage. Emotion is the language of the soul, nudging us to pay attention to our relationship to the world, to people, to God and to ourselves.

In addition to our own internal stimulation, we are stimulated by external sounds and colors, odors and fragrances, varying qualities of air temperature, sizes, shapes and textures as well as magnetic forces emanating from animals, plants, people and even objects in our environment.

It is impossible for us to pay attention with all of our senses to this continual onslaught of sensual stimulation. Our mind helps us to function, moment to moment, by filtering out of our conscious awareness, much of the sensual stimulation we receive. What our mind pays attention to and focuses on determines what we feel now, in the present moment. Our present feelings affect what our mind focuses on and how the world responds to us, now and also in the future.

We are taught to value our mind more than our bodily sensations. We believe our own thoughts as if they were the absolute truth. But each of us has multitudes of varying and even contradictory thoughts every moment throughout the day, every single day we are alive. Which of these many thoughts should we believe? Which of our many thoughts is the truth? Our mind is truly the most powerful creative force in the universe. What we believe will often eventually appear in physical form. We need to begin to carefully choose the thoughts we are willing to allow into our conscious awareness.

We also value words. We often erroneously believe that by talking, by explaining what we are thinking, we will be able to control our world and at the same time create intimate love with our chosen partners. However, often our partners do not appear to listen to the words we so readily express. And our partners' verbal responses are often not the words we would like to hear. In fact, in many relationships, the more words we use, the less intimate we seem to become.

What Is True Intimacy?

What passes for honest, "intimate" communication is often nothing more than an intellectual exercise, devoid of heartfelt emotion. Sometimes we verbally express what we **think** we feel without paying attention to even the most blatant bodily messages. For example, we might say, "I'm not angry," while holding a tight fist and clenching our teeth in suppressed rage. We might say, "Sex is not important to me anymore," whereupon our throat clogs up in an uncontrollable urge to cough. In some cases, we use verbal communication as a way to justify our position, to whitewash our inconsiderate actions, or to purposely intimidate and belittle our "intimate" partners.

True intimacy implies freedom, freedom to reveal our deepest fears, hurts and insecurities as well as our grandest dreams. Intimacy also implies longevity and commitment within an ongoing relationship. Revealing our deepest self to a stranger in a bar, on an airplane, or in a brief sexual liaison, (someone who we will probably never meet again), does not require the soul searching, compassion and responsibility of true intimacy.

Intimacy implies responsibility. In an intimate relationship, we not only express our thoughts and feelings openly and honestly, we also listen to our partner's concerns, absorb the emotional impact of their words, attempt to comprehend the deeper meanings, and take appropriate action as needed to rectify the situation if possible.

In an intimate relationship we feel safe, not because we expect our partner to always treat us with kindness and compassion, but because we know that our partner truly has our own best interests at heart. We feel safe because, over time, we recognize our partner's style of communicating and responding. We appreciate the ways that our partner is courageous and strong when we feel most inadequate and vulnerable. And we feel acknowledged when our partner appreciates us for the ways we are courageous and strong when our partner feels inadequate and vulnerable.

Intimacy implies a shared history. We understand without words. We are able to be our most natural self, freely talking in our own way or comfortably remaining silent. An intimate relationship allows us to face our self and each other, without the need to hide or pretend. Over time we discover and uncover more and more about our own self in relationship and about our partner.

We know a lot more than most of us realize about people we are meeting for the first time, even and especially before any words are spoken. In fact, words often confuse our original and accurate perceptions, causing us to disregard or doubt what our senses have revealed to us. Discover how much you already know about people you may have never met.

What Do You Know About Others?

On the street, on public transportation, at a restaurant or party, even at your office, observe people you have never met before. Observe the expression on their faces. Gaze into their eyes. Pay attention to their nonverbal behavior, physical appearance, body posturing, and emotional attitude. Listen carefully to not only their words, but the tone and quality of their voices. Compare people to each other. Who appears to be more or less confident, happy, depressed, lonely, angry, or insecure? Who appears to be satisfied with their self and who seems to be pretending and hiding some deep insecurity?

Sometimes our perceptions are wrong or slightly off, but more often than not, we are right on target. How is that possible, if we have not engaged in lengthy conversations and we know nothing about this person's personal history? Without words, how do we know another person?

What Does Your Intuitive Sense Reveal To You?

One major way that we know another is through our five senses. We see, hear, smell, touch, and sometimes even taste, the people closest to us. We learn a lot about others through our five senses. But there is something so evident that most of us do not realize it is so. We know others through our own mind as we receive their thoughts. Thoughts are powerful. They actually have form and substance. If we pay attention, we can sometimes truly read another's thoughts. We know how they feel by the expression on their face, the intensity in their eyes, and the way they carry their body.

We also have an intuitive sense. When we breathe deeply, relax our body, and calm the restless scanning of our perpetually thinking mind, we come to a place of knowing. We have a sense that something or someone is good for us, dangerous, confusing, difficult to understand, or should be avoided.

Blocking Your Senses To Reveal More

There is something more, something indefinable, lying beneath, behind, or between our subtle thoughts, our five physical senses, and our intuitive sixth sense. We might call this place our spiritual sense. This is a place where we connect with all the knowledge that ever was, is or will be. This is the place from which so-called creative genius are able to make their discoveries and create their masterpieces. So often we hear them say, "I didn't create.... It was as if it was dictated to me...." Blocking our physical senses allows us to tap into our spiritual sense, to locate that quiet place within, that place of peace and calm, that place of universal energy, that we share with everyone and everything that exists.

BLOCK YOUR SIGHT

Close Your Eyes.

Place a blindfold or your palms gently against your upper cheek bones, cupping your eyes closed.

Notice how that is for you to close your eyes.

Observe your inner sight. What do you see?

How do you feel?

Safe, secure, calm, relaxed….

Afraid, anxious, isolated, angry, insecure....

Begin to walk around the room with the blindfold or your palms securely blocking any light from entering your eyes.

Notice how you feel walking around indoors in a familiar room without seeing.

Walk outside into the hallway of your apartment building or onto your front lawn or back yard if you live in a house or condo. Remember to keep your vision blocked.

Notice how you feel walking around outside of your home without seeing.

Open Your Eyes.

View the world around you with new eyes, soft eyes, beginner's eyes, as if you are seeing everything for the very first time.

What do your eyes notice first?

Focus on one object, person, plant or animal at a time. Observe the shapes and colors, textures and designs, movement or stillness, warmth or coldness, or other qualities.

It has been said that our eyes are the windows to our soul. Through our eyes we contact the world. Our eyes observe the wondrous beauty of nature (mountains, oceans, sunrise, sunset, rainbows, flowers, animals) and the monuments of human creation (buildings, cars, computers, airplanes). Through our peripheral vision, we anticipate movement, as in sports, or spot approaching danger. During war, in the midst of battle, some soldiers claim they were actually able to see and dodge bullets coming at them from the front, side, and even behind their backs. Time seemed to slow down. The bullets appeared to be moving in slow motion. In an intense state of fear, as in war or other trauma or when one or more of our senses are blocked or damaged, our working senses may become more acute. We can see, hear, and feel things we would not ordinarily be able to sense.

BLOCK YOUR HEARING

Close Your Ears.

Place ear plugs, cotton, or your index fingers in your ears, your palms resting on your cheeks.

Notice how that is for you to block out external sound.

Listen to your own inner sound. What do you hear?

How do you feel?

Safe, secure, calm, relaxed....

Afraid, anxious, isolated, angry, insecure....

Begin to walk around the room with your ears blocked.

Notice how you feel walking around indoors in a familiar room without hearing.

Walk outside into the hallway of your apartment building or onto your front lawn or back yard if you live in a house or condo. Remember to keep your hearing blocked.

Notice how you feel walking around outside of your home without hearing.

Open Your Ears.

Listen to the world around you with new ears, beginner's ears, as if you are listening to everything for the very first time.

What do your ears notice first?

Focus on one sound at a time. Observe the volume, amplitude, texture, speed, vibration, movement, loudness or softness, or other qualities of each sound..

Sound warns us of imminent danger or the promise of excitement. The sound of a mother's heartbeat comforts her baby and lulls it to sleep. The sound of a purring cat calms us, causing us to smile, or startles us if we're afraid of cats. A barking dog protects us if we are its owner or frightens us if we are about to be attacked. Our lover's voice can thrill us with passionate sentiment or repel us after an unsettling argument.

The sound of music can have profound healing effects upon our physiological functions. In the best selling book, *Sounds of Healing: A Physician Reveals the Therapeutic Power of Sound, Voice, and Music,* pp. 80-82, the author, Mitchell Gaynor, summarizes the findings of numerous studies about the effects of music:

- Reduced anxiety, heart and respiratory rates in patients who had suffered recent heart attacks.
- Reduced cardiac complications among patients who had been recently admitted to a coronary care unit after suffering heart attacks.
- Lowered systolic blood pressure in nine subjects who listened to two albums of music which had average beats of fewer than 55 hertz, the rate at which a sound wave vibrates.

- Decreased systolic and diastolic blood pressure as much as five points and heart rate as many as four to five beats per minute in subjects who listened to recordings of various musical styles.
- Too much noise, setting off the fight or flight response, can increase blood pressure by as much as 10 percent.
- Reduced blood pressure, heart rate, and noise sensitivity in heart surgery patients who listen to music during the first day after surgery.
- Increased immune cell messengers, levels of interleukin-1, by 12.5-14 percent when subjects listened to music that they liked for fifteen-minute periods.
- Decreased levels of stress hormones, cortisol and ACTH, in patients who listened to music while undergoing gastroscopy (insertion of a probe through the mouth and into the stomach).
- Boost in natural opiates, endorphins, resulting in feelings of euphoria, among subjects who listened to various kinds of music.

What is our world like when we have difficulty hearing or are completely unable to hear sounds? Noted feminist physician, Dr. Christiane Northrup, cites studies about hearing loss in middle aged men. For some reason, they are unable to hear sounds specifically within the speaking range of their long time spouses. Imagine the damaging effect this specific hearing loss might have upon their most intimate relationships, the misunderstandings and hurt feelings that might result.

If we begin to lose our hearing, at first, perhaps, we might feel frustrated as we struggle to comprehend what others are saying. People might become impatient as they are forced to repeat their words, sometimes many times. We might gradually lose interest in socializing with others. Even the most ordinary, simple activities, like talking on the phone, watching TV, going to a movie, dancing, or listening to music, can become stressful and unpleasant experiences. Walking on a busy street or driving a car can become dangerous if we cannot hear sounds that might prevent an accident. If we are wearing a hearing aid, we may be jarred or even pained by the static of background sounds.

If we do not wallow in self-pity or become increasingly reclusive, we may discover life has something much more to offer. When we cannot hear, our other senses may become more acute. We can use our sense of sight to read lips, to observe facial expressions and body movements of others, and also to enjoy the beauty of the world around us. Our sense of taste and smell and touch may intensify. We may have to slow down, to pay attention in the moment. And we can tune out the world whenever we choose.

BLOCK YOUR SENSE OF SMELL

Block Your Sense of Smell

Place a nose clip or the thumb and index finger of your dominant hand on either side of your nose.

Press your nostrils closed.

Notice how it is for you to block out the sense of smell. Observe the effect upon your throat. Notice your natural and immediate need to swallow.

How is that for you to breathe only through your mouth?

Pay attention to your own inner scent. What do you smell?

How do you feel?

Safe, secure, calm, relaxed....

Afraid, anxious, isolated, angry, insecure....

Begin to walk around the room with your nostrils blocked.

Notice how you feel walking around indoors in a familiar room without smelling.

Walk outside into the hallway of your apartment building or onto your front lawn or back yard if you live in a house or condo. Remember to keep your nostrils blocked.

Notice how you feel walking around outside of your home without smelling.

Open Your Sense of Smell.

Smell the world around you with a new nose, beginner's nose, as if you are smelling everything for the very first time.

What do smell first?

Being able to smell will probably save our life many times. Our nose alerts us to the noxious gas of something burning, the unpleasant odor of moldy food, the stench of filth. Our sense of smell also detects our favorite food cooking, the personal scent of our lover or children, perfume fragrances, and the elements of our natural environment: flowers, grass, trees, the ocean, a gentle breeze.

Each of us has a dominant nostril, the same side as our dominant hand, because of greater nerve sensitivity on that side. A healthy person may be able to detect from 10,000 to 30,000 different scents. Yet, each of us has our own unique scent preferences, based upon our society, culture, ethnic group, experiences, memories, or part of the world we live in.

Our ability to perceive odors seems to peak at around age 40, although studies claim it may decline as early as age 20 in some people. Smoking seriously impairs our sense of smell by actually paralyzing the tiny cilia inside the nasal passages. One out of every 20 head injured people describes losing a sense of smell and/or taste. Even a seemingly mild concussion can affect taste and smell sensibility.

Approximately 4 million Americans have problems with their sense of smell and/or taste, not related to aging. Most complain about a total lack of smell (anosmia) or unusual smells (phantosmia). Half of those over 65 and 3/4 of those over 80 have a reduced ability to smell (called hyposmia).

If we are constantly or repeatedly exposed to an odor, we tend to adapt to it, that is, our ability to perceive the odor declines. This lowered sensitivity can persist for as long as three weeks after the odor is removed. However, studies show we are more likely to adapt to the same, identical odor if we believe it is a natural substance rather than a harmful chemical. From the moment of birth, a baby recognizes the scent of its mother, especially if nursed. The baby will stop crying if the mother enters the room, even if the mother is beyond the baby's periphery of sight.

Memories triggered by an odor tend to be more emotionally intense than other sensory cues. Some of the worst memories of war-traumatized, bombing-victims, or sexual abuse victims, are caused by their sense of smell. The scent of burning chemicals, body perspiration, or ejaculated semen can cause a previously traumatized person to instantly have a bodily re-experiencing of the trauma. On the other hand, the aroma of freshly baked cookies, pumpkin pie or an oven roast can warm an adult or elderly person's heart, instantly bringing their memory back to an emotionally comforting, happy time in their childhood.

Dr. Alan R. Hirsch, M.D., author of *Scentsational Sex* (April, 1998), conducted studies to discover what particular scents caused sexual arousal in men and in women. For men, the scent of a combination of lavender and pumpkin pie showed the greatest measurable arousal, increased blood flow to the penis, while licorice and doughnuts as well as cinnamon buns also had a stimulating effect. But arousal in men increased in response to every odor tested. Not so for women. Arousal for women, measured by increased vaginal blood flow, was highest in response to the scent of Good and Plenty, licorice candy, or licorice Allsorts and cucumber combined, but was also affected by a combination of lavender and pumpkin pie. However, women showed negative responses to several odors, including cherry, charcoal barbecue smoke, and male cologne. Scientists are beginning to find evidence that we may also be aroused or turned off by pheromones, the natural scent or chemicals released by our human partners.

BLOCK YOUR SENSE OF TASTE

Block Your Sense of Taste.

Place your thumbs below and the rest of your fingers above your lips, keeping your mouth closed.

Notice how that is for you to block out external taste.

Notice how that is for you to breathe only through your nose.

Pay attention to your own inner taste. What do you taste?

How do you feel?

Safe, secure, calm, relaxed....

Afraid, anxious, isolated, angry, insecure....

Remember a time when you had a bad cold or flu and were unable to smell or taste food. Remember a time when your stomach felt full or you felt slightly nauseous and were unable to enjoy the sight or taste of food that you usually love.

How does it feel to be unable to taste?

Open Your Sense of Taste.

Taste the world around you with a new tongue, beginner's tongue, as if you are tasting everything for the very first time.

What do taste first?

Imagine the subtle or strong taste as you kiss your pet, your child's cheek, your spouse's lips or as you bite into a juicy apple, a tart lemon, a cube of sugar, ice cream covered with hot melted fudge, mashed potatoes, crunchy almonds, a slice of gooey pizza, or any of your favorite foods.

'It's a matter of taste' may be more true than we have ever realized. The French expression, "chacun a son gout" (to each his own taste), describes it well. Humans are, in fact, genetically, culturally and individually different in their ability to perceive food flavors. Scientists have categorized people into supertasters, tasters, and nontasters, based on the number of fungiform papillae, the structures that hold the taste buds, on their tongues. About 25% of the population appear to be supertasters, 25% nontasters, and 50% tasters. Women are more likely to be supertasters, especially when estrogen is at its highest (ovulation, pregnancy). Supertasters tend to be more sensitive to a bitter compound in broccoli and other vegetables or the bitter aftertaste of artificial sweeteners. Nontasters appear to barely perceive these bitter flavors.

Hormonal levels can alter our sense of taste. Estrogen seems to increase taste sensitivity. Pregnant women are notorious for having intense food cravings, often for such unlikely foods as pickles and ice cream, combinations that they would find unpleasant at any other time. During ovulation, women's taste sensitivity is also enhanced.

Taste buds are not only on the tongue, but also scattered on the roof of the mouth, inside the cheeks, even in the throat. Complex interactions occur within and among the taste buds - each filled with nerve fibers. Thus we are able to differentiate among the four basic flavors - sweet, sour, bitter, and salty. The burn of spicy foods is not a flavor in itself; instead of stimulating the taste buds, it activates the bundle of nerves that wrap around each taste bud. Other taste sensations include, metallic, alkaline, and umami, which is the taste of glutamate, as found in MSG (monosodium glutamate).

Taste is not limited only to the sensory perceptions of taste buds. Taste and olfactory sensations combine to determine how people enjoy food. Scientists have coined the term, "mouthsense" to describe this phenomenon. Limiting the foods we eat does not enhance their taste. In fact, our appreciation of food tends to increase when the sense of taste is surprised and challenged. Indeed, "variety is the spice of life."

Another factor in the sense of taste is the trigeminal system, branches of nerves connecting the brain to the nose and the mouth. These nerves detect irritants such as hot chilies, black pepper, coolness of mint, and carbonation in beverages. The texture of food and its visual appearance also affect taste. Hot food gives off more vapor, increasing the intensity of sweet or bitter flavors; cold seems to reduce the impact of these flavors. Sour and salty foods do not seem to be as influenced by temperature.

Most taste preferences are learned. We can educate our self, through careful study and practice, to discern the unique qualities of various foods. Overcoming our initial aversion to the bitter taste, some of us learn to love the flavor of coffee. Wine connoisseurs are able to distinguish the unique taste of different wines, while gourmet chefs use specific spices to create extraordinary taste sensations for our palates.

Our sense of taste is strongly influenced by our sense of smell. In fact, when we are hungry, our sense of smell intensifies. Detecting the aroma of our favorite foods will stimulate our salivary glands. Studies show that people have **lost weight** merely by smelling their favorite foods. Having their olfactory senses stimulated helped them to overcome their craving, without putting any food into their mouth.

Taste sensitivity and the number of taste buds do not decrease with age. Decreased taste sensitivity may be due to memory loss, changes in the brain's perception of tastes, or chronic illness, rather than to changes in the taste buds. However, the sense of smell, which affects enjoyment of different foods, does tend to diminish with age. Studies show that 50% of people over age 65 and 75% of those over age 80, have a reduced ability to smell. One way to compensate for any loss of taste sensitivity is to eat foods with contrasting textures, temperatures, colors, and flavors. How intricate and delicate is our brain wiring for the sense of taste!

BLOCK YOUR SENSE OF TOUCH

Block Your Sense of Touch.

Close your eyes.

Put on a pair of rubber gloves, the thicker the better.

Touch some different household items, a cup, a spoon, a hairbrush.

Imagine you have lost your sense of touch.

What would you miss touching?

What problems or dangers might this cause for you?

Open Your Sense of Touch.

> *Touch the world around you with new hands, beginner's hands, as if you are touching everything for the very first time.*

Touch one object, person, plant or animal at a time. Observe the subtle and strong qualities, varying temperatures and sensations you feel as you touch various textures, fabrics.

Wrapping around our entire body, our skin is the largest and most essential sense organ. If we cannot see, hear speak, taste or smell, we can still survive. But without our skin, our body will cease to exist. Protecting our body structures and internal organs, our skin continually sends messages from the external world directly to our brain and bodily cells. Our skin reflects our age, height, weight, and our state of physical, mental, emotional and even spiritual health or illness. No magical facial surgery can completely mask our inner state.

Touch, even the mere intention to touch, can affect the health, resiliency, texture and responsiveness of our skin and internal organs. How our skin responds to touch is determined by many factors: our genes, gender, health, previous touch experiences, pain threshold, perceptions, beliefs, and memories. Even a light touch on the surface of our skin can have a profound effect: pleasure, pain, irritation, or ticklishness. Each of us responds very differently to touch and we respond differently to the same type of touch at different times and with different people.

Studies show that severe deprivation of touch in the early years can lead to death or lifelong mental retardation. A startling discovery was made in Lebanon in the 1960's when foundlings, infants living at an orphanage, The Crêche, were finally allowed to be legally adopted. Until that point, it was widely believed that these children were mentally deficient and would never develop normal intelligence. To everyone's surprise, those foundlings adopted before 2 years of age developed normal I.Q.'s. Those adopted after age two, maintained some mental retardation, but their intellect level improved somewhat over time. Those foundlings who remained at The Crêche failed to develop normal intelligence because they were deprived of sensory stimulation, including touch.

Recent research indicates that intentional, massaging touch (even 15 minutes, 3 times a week) improves vital signs, activity level and growth of infants, lessens anxiety in adults, and alleviates depression in the elderly. A noted neuroscientist, Dr. James Prescott, suggests that lack of touch and bodily pleasure in the early years is the principle cause of human violence. Harry Harlow's experiments in the 1960's and 1970's showed that infant monkeys deprived of a warm, soft, comforting mother's touch developed inadequate social and sexual skills for their entire lives.

Touch heals. Touch also hurts. And the absence of touch can cause irreversible harm. How do we treat for lack of touch, memories of painful or abusive touch, or our lifelong need to be touched, and hugged and held? Touch can be introduced to a touch aversive person – slowly and very carefully, in a safe and trusting environment, with a safe and trusted person with a lot of patience and compassionn, over a very long period of time.

BLOCK ALL YOUR SENSES

Cover your eyes, with a blindfold, a scarf, or with your hands.

Put ear plugs, cotton or your index fingers into your ears.

Use a nose clip or press your nostrils closed using your middle fingers.

Close your mouth.

Hold your breath.

Notice how that is for you to block off all your senses and hold your breath.

How do you feel?

Open your mouth slightly to allow yourself to breathe through your mouth, keeping all of your other senses blocked.

Listen to your own internal sounds.

Observe the colors, shapes or visions that appear in your inner sight.

Watch your thoughts as they come and go.

Observe your own internal tastes and smells.

Imagine the sensation of touching and being touched.

Notice how you feel in your body now.

GO ON A SENSUAL HOLIDAY

OPEN ALL YOUR SENSES

Plan to give yourself a sensual bonanza.

Explore all your senses at once.

Consciously use your eyes to watch, observe and soak in everything around you: shapes,

colors, energetic fields, dust particles, body language, facial expressions.

Plan to go to movies, theatre, ballet, sports events, art galleries, horse races, and even while on your computer – pay attention to the sights you see.

Consciously listen to even the most subtle sounds and words with both ears.

Listen to different types of music: vocal, instrumental and electronic.

Listen to different people, children, teenagers, adults, talking, lecturing, laughing, crying, giggling, fighting and playing.

Consciously smell everything and everyone.

Smell the flowers on the table at a restaurant or along your walking path.

Smell the wine or coffee, appetizer, entrée and dessert, before eating.

Smell the food cooking at home.

Smell the food as you bite into each and every morsel.

Smell your pets, your children, your partner, and other people nearby.

Consciously taste a wide variety of foods, cooked in different ways.

Chew slowly.

Attempt to distinguish each and every spice and flavor.

Notice in what part of your mouth you actually taste the food.

Consciously touch and feel the texture, shape, and temperature of objects, nature and people in your environment (being ethically and socially appropriate).

Touch people.

Hug people, your intimate partner, your children, your elderly relatives,your friends and acquaintances.

Allow yourself to be touched and hugged.

Experience what it is like to live in a totally sensational world! Experience what it is like to block all your senses. No longer aware of sensations, discover the nonphysical, nonmaterial part of yourself, the part that knows and connects with everyone and everything, the part that knows God. Allow your senses to flood back into your life, in every moment, thoughts at bay, judgments gone, aware of only pure, ever-present, sensation. Imagine being with your lover, speaking to your co-workers, standing up for your rights, putting your children to sleep, in that sensational state of heightened awareness of your mind, body and spirit and the mind, body and spirit of others.

TOUCHING MATTERS

THE PROFOUND EFFECTS

OF TOUCH AND BODY THERAPY

CHAPTER 3

TOUCHING MATTERS

THE PROFOUND EFFECTS OF TOUCH AND BODY THERAPY

Touch Me

Your gentle soothing hand
Calms and comforts me
Relieves
My inner longing
I feel safe, secure, connected
Your touch reminds me
I am not alone
I can let go of control
And feel
All there is to feel
Allowing myself to finally be
Me

Touch Is Powerful

Touch is powerful. Our sense of self, ability to love, attractiveness to others, and sexual passion, often hinges upon the way we touch and respond to touch. Sexual desire may be either stimulated or suppressed by the mere hint of an impending touch. With harsh or abusive touch, we tend to constrict our body, repress our feelings and become less receptive to love. Loving touch assists us to release painful memories and open our heart to others. Touching our self brings a profound sense of inner peace, self-acceptance and self-love.

Research indicates that touch promotes health, healing and general well-being, from

pregnancy and birth to every stage of development throughout life. Teachers, psychotherapists, and even waiters arc evaluated as more caring, knowledgeable and competent when they casually touch their students, clients, or customers in a non-threatening, non-sexual way. Even in this litigious and touch aversive climate of today's society, caring touch brings us closer to one another.

Touch In Psychotherapy

Research indicates that touch in psychotherapy can be helpful, powerful or destructive depending upon the way it is used, the therapist's intention and the client's perceptions. Undergraduate and graduate college students described a counselor (male or female) they observed touching a client, as more caring than the counselor who did not touch (Driscoll, 1986). Patients' experiences with touch in therapy indicated that touch enhanced self-esteem and fostered a bond that allowed for greater trust, openness and acceptance. Contrary to what most of us might expect, sexual abuse survivors rated therapist touch significantly more positively than did non survivors, emphasizing trust and learning about boundaries in relationships (Horton, 1994). Touch can assist therapists to tap into their clients' deep emotional processes, assisting patients to break unhealthy relationship bonds (Cronise, 1993).

Touch can either assist or interfere with the psychotherapeutic process. Motivations of therapists for touching may include trying to improve physiological functioning, seeking personal gratification of therapist or client, education or interpersonal exploration, somatic/emotional release, sexual and physical gratification, socially appropriate contact, perceived necessity, and intuition (Weisberg, 1992).

Psychotherapy clients found touch in psychotherapy to be beneficial if they were free to talk about the touch, boundaries, and sexual feelings; if they felt control over initiating or sustaining contact; if the touch was not demanded by the therapist; and if the expectations of the therapist for emotional and physical intimacy matched their own reality. Clients felt confused or negative about the touch in psychotherapy if they felt guilty about being angry at their therapist, trapped in having to be close, or were repeating unpleasant childhood dynamics. (Geib,Ph.D., Boston University School of Education, 1982).

Should psychotherapists touch their clients? Yes, perhaps occasionally, to indicate comfort, concern, and compassion. No, in general, unless the psychotherapist can verify years of training, appropriate professional certification and licensure in both touch therapy and therapeutic counseling. Body therapists, on the other hand, who often perform exquisitely intricate body movements, manipulations and muscular tension releases, are not usually trained to deal with emotional issues. Touch within a therapeutic session is extremely sensitive and intimate. Body psychotherapists, certified or licensed as psychotherapists and also certified or licensed in one or more body therapy modalities, are uniquely qualified to introduce touch as an agreed upon component of the therapeutic relationship. Body psychotherapy requires years of training, experience and ongoing supervision.

The Profound Effects of Touch

Touch Research Institute Studies

Touching and being touched has profound healing effects at all ages (from pre-term infants to adolescents, adults and even elderly grandparents) and for a wide variety of ailments and diseases (from asthma, diabetes and fibromyalgia to HIV+ and AIDS. During a one-year sabbatical from my professorship in 1995, I took a brief training at the Touch Research Institute at Jackson Memorial Hospital, Miami, Florida, with Dr. Tiffany Field, psychologist and leading touch therapy researcher in the world. Touch Research Institute studies have been conducted worldwide, for many years, utilizing a simple protocol, easily replicated by other researchers. Subjects receive 15-30 minute massage sessions, 2 times per week for 5 weeks. Control groups receive standard nursing treatment, TENS (electrical stimulation), SHAM TENS (use of the TENS machine without electrical stimulation), or progressive relaxation. Although the TENS treatment and progressive relaxation have some positive effects, massage has more significant and long-lasting effects.

What follows is an overview of the types of studies conducted at the Touch Research Institute and the powerful results attained by a minimal amount of touch (15-30 minutes, 2 times per week).

Studies of **preterm newborns**, suggest that infants who are touched at regular intervals, compared to those who are not touched, gain more weight, become more responsive, are discharged from the hospital several days earlier, and upon follow-up 8 months later, are still showing greater weight gain, mental and motor development. **Cocaine-exposed** and **HIV-exposed newborns** who receive touch exhibit increased weight, reduced stress levels, and better performance on the Brazleton Newborn Scale, particularly motor development.

Infants who are touched have greater daily weight gain, more organized sleep/wake behaviors, less fussiness, improved sociability, greater interaction with others, and lower cortisol and norepinephrine indicating lower stress levels and increased serotonin which suggests less depression.

Preschool children who receive massage fall asleep sooner, have more restful nap periods, and have decreased activity levels. For **autistic children**, touch sensitivity, attention to sounds, off-task classroom behavior decrease while relatedness to teacher increases, after receiving massage. **Children who are touched after surviving a natural disaster** show decreased anxiety, depression and cortisol levels. **Diabetic childrens'** glucose levels decrease to the normal range while **asthmatic children** exhibit increased peak air flow, fewer asthma attacks, and less anxiety and depression after being touched. **Juvenile rheumatoid arthritic children** experience lower anxiety and cortisol levels and less pain. Massage therapy reduces agitation and pain levels before debridement in **children with severe burns.**

Adolescent studies show that **anorexic and bulimic girls** have improved body image and decreased depression and anxiety symptoms when touched. Massage therapy decreases anxiety and pain, reduces the length of labor and the need for medication for **teenage mothers in childbirth** and decreases depression and anxiety in **depressed teenage mothers**.

And for the **elderly**, studies indicate that **grandparent volunteers** report less anxiety, fewer depressive symptoms, improved mood, fewer doctor visits, improved lifestyle, decreased pulse rate and improved self-esteem, after giving massage to infants. These effects were stronger after giving than after receiving massages.

For adults, **job performance** studies indicate that after receiving massage, participants experience increased alertness, faster completion of math problems with 50% less errors and lower anxiety levels. Hospital staff members show significantly reduced anxiety, depression and fatigue. **Fibromyalgia** patients experience decreased pain levels, improved sleep patterns, decreased fatigue, anxiety, depression and cortisol levels while chronic fatigue syndrome patients have shown reduced fatigue related symptoms, including emotional stress, somatic symptoms, depression and difficulty sleeping. **Rape and spouse abuse victims** exhibit a decreased aversion to touch, decreased anxiety, depression and cortisol levels.

Dr. Tiffany Field's studies involve mostly traditional massage. She has created a network of franchised Touch Research centers, repeating similar research protocols, throughout the United States and in Europe. However, there are a wide variety of other methods and techniques that utilize touch, from painful, invasive, deep tissue work to gentle, balancing and even lighter energetic techniques. Many studies on other forms of body therapy, until recently, have been conducted in Europe within traditional medical and psychological settings.

The National Institutes for Health, Office of Alternative and Complementary Medicine began awarding research grants in 1993. Several of the grants studied the effects of various body therapies. That same year The American Massage Therapy Association Foundation began offering research grants. The Upledger Institute Healthplex Center, in Palm Beach Gardens, Florida, has been conducting research for years on the use of craniosacral therapy and somatoemotional release to improve conscious awareness of brain function, posttraumatic stress disorder and the bioelectric transference between patient and therapist during therapeutic sessions. Research on body therapy is still in the early stages, but results so far have been quite promising.

Body Therapy
Which One is Right for You?

Although, Touch Research Institute studies have shown beyond a reasonable doubt that massage heals, massage is only one style of body therapy. Most of us are not aware that there are as many ways to touch as there are people to develop methods. Body therapy includes many different styles of touch, movement, and body awareness exercises. Some methods involve direct contact with the skin, some realign the structure of the body, some re-balance the craniosacral rhythm or the meridian system, while others affect the aura or energetic field. A strict code of ethics, developed and established by the national certifying or licensing board or the specialized certification program, is an essential component of body therapy training. Body therapy does not and should not involve sexual contact of any kind and is not for the purpose of sexual release. However, the resulting muscular relaxation and energetic re-balancing of the body often leads to greater ease and pleasure in all aspect of life, including intimate sexual relations.

To help determine which techniques resonate with our own personal bodily needs, each of the various body therapy methods have been classified within seven categories. These categories are not exclusive. Some methods may fit into more than one category. For each descriptive category, a brief summary is presented. For books, videos, web sites, training programs, and how to locate a qualified practitioner of a specific modality in your area, refer to the Appendices at the end of this book.

1. Swedish Massage/Therapeutic Massage
2. Contemporary Western Massage and Body Therapy
3. Structural, Functional, Movement, Alignment Body Therapy
4. Asian Body Therapy
5. Energetic Body Therapy
6. Somatic and Expressive Arts Body Therapy
7. Body Psychotherapy.

Swedish Massage
Traditional Massage Therapy

Probably the most well known, the most thoroughly researched, and one of the few licensed methods of touch therapy in this country, is Swedish Massage or Massage Therapy. In a typical session, the client usually lies on a massage table, totally unclothed, wearing undergarments, or wearing shorts and a tee shirt. Most of the client's body is comfortably draped in sheets and towels, with only the body part being massaged left uncovered. With a combination of oils or creams, herbal and aromatic essences, music, soft lighting, and sometimes colored lights, the massage therapist uses five basic massage strokes (effleurage, petrissage, friction, tapotement, vibration) directly upon the client's skin. The pressure used in the strokes should vary according to the client's preferences.

The goal of massage therapy is to relax the mind and body, relieve symptoms of pain or stress, and sometimes to assist clients to create a healthier, more holistic lifestyle which includes improving diet, exercise, rest and sleep habits. Massage is generally accessible and affordable. Many massage schools have clinics in which advanced students give a series of massages at very reduced rates. The profession of massage therapy has been rapidly gaining respect through state licensing, national certifications, national accreditation of training programs and schools, insurance coverage, and official recognition as an important healing modality at the Olympics.

Contemporary Western Massage and Bodywork

Contemporary Western Massage and Bodywork includes body therapy methods and techniques that alleviate muscular tension, painful nerve constrictions, poor circulation, and chronic aches and pains caused by stress, overwork, overexertion, athletic and other injuries, pregnancy, hormonal imbalances, and illnesses. Expanding upon the practice of Traditional Massage Therapy, these methods include the use of water, ice and heat, massage in the work place or outdoors, massage focused on body parts injured from accidents and diseases, gentle sensual massage, massage to improve athletic performance and to heal athletic injuries, as well as massage specially geared for pregnancy, for infants, and even for animals.

Aquassage/Hydrotherapy (Ice & Heat)
Animal Massage
Chair Massage
Esalen Massage

Infant Massage
Kripalu Bodywork
Medical Massage
Myotherapy
On-Site Massage
Pregnancy Massage
Pfrimmer Deep Muscle Therapy
Sports Massage
Watsu (Water Massage)

Structural/Functional Movement/Integration

Structural, Functional, Movement Integration body therapy methods include techniques to improve body alignment, organ functioning, flexibility of movement, and integration of the body as a holographic system. These methods may involve actual re-sculpting of the connective tissue, improved flow of cerebrospinal fluid, lymph drainage, realignment of vertebrae, release of muscle, nerve and membrane restrictions, inhibition of habitual posture patterns, stimulation of trigger points and reflexes to specific organs, or simply guiding the body to move in an easier, more graceful manner.

Alexander Technique
Applied Kinesiology
Aston-Patterning
Bindegewebsmassage/Connective Tissue
Body Logic
Bowen Method
Chiropractic

Craniosacral
Feldenkrais
Hellerwork
Holotropic Breathwork
Kurashova Method Russian Massage
Laban Movement Analysis
Lomi Lomi
Looyenwork
Manual Lymph Drainage
Mensendiek System
Myofascial Release
Network Chiropractic
Neuromuscular
Osteopathy
Physiatry
Physical Therapy
Rebirthing
Reflexology
Rolfing
Strain/Counterstrain
Touch For Health
Trager & Mentastics
Trigger Point Therapy
Visceral Manipulation

Asian Bodywork

Asian Bodywork includes body therapy methods and techniques originating throughout Asia, mostly derived from traditional Chinese medicine theory. This theory describes the health of the body in terms of the five basic elements (fire, water, earth, metal, and wood) or the functioning of the 12 pairs of primary meridians (lung, large intestine, stomach, spleen, heart, small intestine, bladder, kidney, pericardium or heart constrictor, triple heater, gall bladder, and liver) and the 8 extraordinary meridians (including conception vessel and governing vessel which run directly down the center line of the body in the front and back respectively).

Most of these methods utilize the therapist's fingers and hands, although some techniques use the therapist's shoulders, elbows, knees, and even feet. Acupuncture involves insertion of very fine needles into precise meridian locations. Therapists may determine which meridians to treat by utilizing various diagnostic methods, including differentiating among the 12 pulses in the wrist, examining the qualities of the organs represented on the hara (abdominal area), and observing the client's eyes, ears, throat and tongue.

Some methods involve extensive stretching and twisting movements, an actual physical workout for both the therapist and client. Other methods are more gentle, focusing on controlling and expanding the breath or holding various bodily positions, not unlike yoga postures. The goal of these methods is to release restrictions in the flow of energy or chi throughout the body.

Acupressure
Acupuncture
Amma (Anma)
Amma Therapy
Chi Gong (Qi Gong) (Chi Kung)
Chun Do Sun Bup
Do-In
Jin Shin Do Bodymind Acupressure
Jin Shin Jyutsu
Lomi Lomi
Ohashiatsu
Thai Massagge
Tuina

Energetic Bodywork

Energetic bodywork includes body therapy methods and techniques from healers around the world, focusing on the energetic fields within and surrounding our bodies. These methods range from direct contact on the skin, to indirect contact an inch to a foot or more above the body, to distant indirect contact from another room, another city, or anywhere on the planet. Training in these methods may be simple or complex, requiring anywhere from a basic one-weekend training to an ongoing series of structured lessons for one to three years or longer. Some methods may involve an initiation process, transferring of healing potential from teacher to student, while other methods teach students to become attuned to their own natural healing potential.

Access
Aura Balancing
Barbara Brennan School
Chakra Healing
Chi Self Massage
Energy Balancing
Intuitive Medicine
Mariel
Multiincarnational Recall
Emotional Body Balancing
Polarity Therapy
Pranic Healing
Radiance Technique
Reiki
Seven Rays
Shamanism
Therapeutic Touch
Zero Balancing

Somatic and Expressive Arts Therapies

Somatic and expressive arts therapies include body-centered therapies and activities that may or may not involve actual touch. Through movement, dance, sports, yoga postures, martial arts, dramatic performances, artistic expression, visualization, as well as through touch, our bodies may express feelings that have previously been unavailable to our conscious minds. Some somatic and expressive arts therapists are trained artists (musicians, singers, actors, dancers, and artists). Others received their major training in one or more body therapy methods. Although some somatic and expressive arts therapists have been educated in graduate academic programs (music therapy, dance therapy, art therapy), many have not received psychotherapy training. Clients would be well advised to seek the assistance of a qualified psychotherapist, to help them assimilate into their daily lives, the powerful emotional experiences that may result from this type of therapy.

Art Therapy
Biofeedback
Dance Therapy
Deep Emotional Release Work
EMDR (Eye Movement Desensitization Reprocessing)
Hypnotherapy
Iridology
Martial Arts
Movement Therapy
Music Therapy
Ortho-Bionomy
Phoenix Rising Yoga Therapy
Pilates Method
Primal Therapy
Primal Integration
Process Acupressure
Psychodrama
Somatoemotional Release
Sports And Exercise
Thought Field Therapy
Visualization

When our bodies move, are touched directly, indirectly or even from a great distance, our emotional equilibrium is often affected. Repressed feelings we didn't even know we had may come bubbling to the surface. Tears, anger, confusion, fear, and childhood memories often emerge unexpectedly.

Many body therapists are highly skilled practitioners. Many are licensed in their state or nationally certified in their specific body therapy modality. However, most do not have adequate, if any, psychotherapy training. Qualified psychotherapists are required to have the following minimal academic credentials:

- Psychiatrist, M.D. degree
- Psychologist, Ph.D. degree
- Clinical Social Worker, M.S.W. degree
- Marriage and Family Therapist, M.A. degree
- Clinical Mental Health Counselor, M.A. degree
- Psychiatric Nurse, R.N. and M.S. degrees.

However, just as qualified body therapists often do not have psychotherapy training, qualified psychotherapists do not usually have adequate, **if any**, body therapy training.

In 1996, The First National Conference on Body Oriented Psychotherapy/The 4th International Congress of Psycho-Corporeal Therapies, met in Beverly, Massachusetts. This coming together of many of the leading body oriented psychotherapists in this country and in the world, led to the creation of the USABP (United States Association for Body Psychotherapy). The first official USABP conference was held in Boulder, Colorado, in June 1998, the second was held in June 2000, and the third is scheduled for 2002. The author of this book, Dr. Erica Goodstone, was one of the original thirteen steering committee members who steered this important organization into the professional status and international recognition it has today.

The goals of this organization are twofold: * to educate the public about this powerful transformative work and * to create ethical guidelines, educational standards, certification and licensing review boards of this burgeoning profession. **Without exception, every person who has combined touch with counseling reports profound and often seemingly miraculous results happening in sessions with their clients.**

Somatic Body Psychotherapy

Body Psychotherapists (sometimes called Body Oriented Psychotherapists or Somatic Body Psychotherapists) are trained and certified in both psychotherapy and body therapy methods or in specific modalities that combine psychotherapy with touch and body awareness. The counseling modalities used in body psychotherapy are similar to those used in traditional talk psychotherapy (psychoanalysis, behavior modification, gestalt therapy, cognitive therapy, even hypnosis). There are many different types of body psychotherapy. Some are very gentle and respectful of the client's needs and boundaries. Other methods are more forceful, focused on breaking through defenses and body armoring. The common element of all body psychotherapy methods is the use of touch and the focus on body awareness. A body psychotherapy session may include guided imagery, focused breathing, role playing, movement, expressive arts, and emotional release while at the same time counseling clients about the psychological underpinnings and current meanings of the issues and emotions that emerge.

Bioenergetic Analysis
Bodymind Centering
Bodynamics

Calatonia and Subtle Touch (Brazilian)
Core Energetics
Focusing
Hakomi Integrative Somatics
Integrative Body Psychotherapy
Lomi School
Organismic Psychotherapy
Pesso Boyden Psychomotor System
Radix
Reichian Therapy
Rosen Method
Rubenfeld Synergy
Somatics
Somatic Psychotherapy Biosynthesis

Touch Is Essential For Living

Of all the five senses, touch is the most essential. We can lose our sight and hearing and ability to speak, yet still find pleasure in the taste and smell of food, the scent of flowers, animals, and people we love, and the sensation of touching and being touched. If we no longer smell or taste our food, we can still derive pleasure from feeling the various textures with our lips, our tongues and our teeth. We can still enjoy touching and being touched.

Without touch, we do not thrive. Babies, adults, and the aged alike, become angry, depressed, despondent, and eventually get sick and die when deprived of touch and sensual stimulation. Humans are communal beings.

We need, desire, and crave contact with each other. People who have lost their mobility have reminded us of the life-saving importance of touch.

Well-known author Helen Keller, blind, deaf and unable to speak from birth, was taught to use her mind, learned to touch and enjoy being touched. She thrived on human contact, without words. Ken Keyes Jr., noted author and workshop leader, without the use of his arms and legs, married and enjoyed touching and being touched throughout his life. After a tragic equestrian accident that left him paralyzed, the popular actor Christopher Reeves, in several intimate TV interviews, tearfully reminded us of the power of touch. His wife stroking his forehead and his son kissing his cheeks kept him connected to feeling human and alive. It is touch that puts Helen Keller, Ken Keyes Jr., Christopher Reeves, and most of us, in contact with our essential humanness and capacity to give and receive love.

The Healing Power of Touch

Touch heals. Touch also hurts. Being touched by someone we love or receiving touch from a skilled and caring body therapist is often a joy. Being touched by someone with an unclear or harmful intention sometimes hurts. Nowadays, touching with even the most honorable intention, has become suspect in this country. In fact, some school districts are taking a very strong stance against teachers who touch students for any reason. Touching a student can be grounds for immediate dismissal. Even among students, if one student claims that touch by another student was inappropriate or abusive, the courts may *now hold the school district responsible. But research about touch in psychotherapy indicates mostly positive effects.

When we are touched, we often feel emotions we have not felt for a long time, as we become more aware of unresolved issues in our lives. When we express our emotions in the presence of a caring and skilled therapist, painful memories emerge, are expressed, and lose their emotional charge. Only then can we begin to enjoy pleasurable experiences and sensations, creating new, positive and pleasant memories.

How Have You Been Touched?

- *How are you touched in your current relationship?*
- *What are your earliest touch memories?*
- *Were you touched frequently, sometimes, or hardly at all?*
- *What was the quality of touch you received: pleasant, unpleasant, gentle, harsh, abusive, intrusive, sensual, sexual, wanted, unwanted?*

How Do You Touch?

- *How do you touch in your current relationship?*
- *What are your earliest memories of touching others?*
- *Did you touch others frequently, sometimes, or hardly at all?*
- *What was the quality of your touch like for others: pleasant, unpleasant, gentle, harsh, abusive, intrusive, sensual, sexual, wanted, unwanted by others?*

TOUCH YOUR BODY

- *What body parts are most sensitive, least sensitive, painful, numb, sensual, pleasurable?*
- *What body parts do you want someone to touch? Why?*
- *What body parts do you want others not to touch? Why not?*

In each of the following touching exercises, notice your thoughts and feelings as you touch each body part. After you become comfortable touching yourself, you can repeat this exercise with a willing partner.

Massage Your Body

Gently and firmly rub, grasp and massage your body, in the following sequence. With your right hand and fingers, massage your left shoulder, upper arm, elbow, forearm, wrist and hand. With your left hand and fingers, massage your right shoulder, upper arm, elbow, forearm, wrist and hand. With both hands massage your lower back, waist, abdomen; upper back and chest, neck and throat. Press your fingers into the base of head and across your entire scalp. Gently rub and caress your temples, ears, chin, jaw, cheeks, forehead and entire face.

Shake and Rock Your Body

Gently and firmly shake and rock your body, in the following sequence: left shoulder, arm and hand; right shoulder, arm and hand; left leg, right leg. Shake your hips from side to side, forward/back, and in circles to the right and circles to the left. Shake your jaw, neck and head. Hold both shoulders and rock yourself like a baby.

Hold Your Body

Rub both hands together to build heat and energy. In a seated position, use both hands to gently hold the following body parts for 30 seconds: Using right palm, hold left shoulder, upper arm, elbow, forearm, wrist, hand. Using left palm, hold right shoulder, upper arm, elbow, forearm, wrist, hand. Place both hands on knees, thighs and then hips.. Place right hand on abdomen and left hand on lower back. Place both hands close together on back of neck, on chin, and then on cheeks. Place right hand on upper chest and left hand on vertebrae in upper back and neck. Place right hand in front of throat and left hand on back of neck. Place right hand on forehead and left hand on base of skull. Place fingertips on eyelids without pressing. Cross arms and place one palm on each shoulder.

TOUCH YOUR PARTNER'S BODY

If you do not have a partner, skip this exercise. You can return to it at some future date with a new partner. If you do have a partner, repeat the previous exercises by taking turns touching your partner and having your partner touch you. Notice your thoughts and feelings, as the toucher or touchee.

Massage Your Partner's Body

Before approaching your partner's body, ask for permission. Throughout this exercise be mindful of your partner's possible sensitivity and self-consciousness. Stop and ask for permission often. If your partner expresses discomfort at any point, remove your hands immediately and only continue with your partner's expressed permission. Now begin to massage your partner's body, gently, firmly, and with utmost respect, in the following sequence. With both hands and fingers, massage your partner's left shoulder, upper arm, elbow, forearm, wrist and hand. Then massage your partner's left shoulder, upper arm, elbow, forearm, wrist and hand. Now, with both hands massage your partner's lower back, waist, abdomen, upper back and chest, neck and throat. Press your fingers into the base of head and across your entire scalp. Gently rub and caress your temples, ears, chin, jaw, cheeks, forehead and entire face.

Shake and Rock Your Partner's Body

With both hands, shake and rock your partner's body, gently and firmly, in the following sequence. Ask your partner to stand. With both hands gently and firmly shake your partner's left shoulder, arm and hand. Now shake your partner's right shoulder, arm and hand. Shake your partner's left leg followed by shaking the right leg. Now, firmly and respectfully, move your partner's hips from side to side, forward/back, and in circles to the right and circles to the left. Gently and firmly move your partner's jaw, neck and head. Wrap both your arms around your partner's upper back and rock gently as if you were holding a tender baby.

Hold Your Partner's Body

Ask your partner to sit with eyes closed. Rub your own hands together to build heat and energy. Place your hands on your partner's body, holding each position for 30 seconds, in the following sequence. Hold your partner's right shoulder, upper arm, elbow, forearm, wrist, and hand. Now hold your partner's left shoulder, upper arm, elbow, forearm, wrist, hand. Place both hands on your partner's feet, ankles, knees, thighs and then hips.. Place your right hand on your partner's abdomen and your left hand on your partner's lower back. Place both hands close together on the back of your partner's neck, on the chin, and then on your partner's cheeks. Place your right hand on your partner's upper chest and your left hand on the vertebrae in the upper back and neck. Place your right hand very lightly in front of your partner's throat and your left hand in back of the neck. Place your right hand on your partner' forehead and your left hand at the base of your partner's skull. Very gently without any pressure place your fingertips on your partner's eyelids. Finish by placing both of your hands firmly on your partner's shoulders.

When you have completed the sequence, repeat this exercise with the receiver becoming the toucher. When you have both been touchers and touchees, spend a few minutes describing what this touching experience has been like for you in both roles.

FOOTNOTES

Chapter 1

1. **Pert, Candace, Ph.D.** ***Molecules of Emotion***
2. **Locke, Steven, M.D. , Ader R, Besedovskhy H, Hall, NR, Solomon, GF, Strom, T. editors (1985).** ***Foundations of Psychoneuroimmunology.*** **Hawthorne, NY: Aldine Publishing Co.**

3. **Reich, Wilhelm, Carfagno, Vincent R., Translator. (1973) *The Function of the Orgasm: Discovery of the Orgone.* NY: Farrar, Straus and Giroux.**

Chapter 2

1. **Wayne, Dennis (1973). *Children of the Creche.* New York. Appleton-Century-Crofts.**
2. **Gaynor, Mitchell. (June 1999) *Sounds of Healing: A Physician Reveals the Therapeutic Power of Sound, Voice, and Music*. NY: Broadway Books**
3. **Christiane Northrup (2006) *The Wisdom of Menopause: Creating Physical and Emotional Health and Healing During the Change.* NY: Bantam Books.**
4. **Alan R. Hirsch, M.D. (April, 1998) *Scentsational Sex: The Secret to Using Aroma for Arousal.* Element Books**
5. **Prescott, James. *How Culture Shapes the Developing Brain and the Future of Humanity.* (March 2004). Byron Child/Kindred, Issue 9.**
6. **Harlow, Harry, F. M.D. R "Development of affection in primates. Pp/ 157-166 in: E. L. Bliss, Ed. (1962) *Roots of Behavior*. NY: Harper.**

Chapter 3

1. **http://www.miami.edu/touch-research/ (Field, Tiffany, Touch Research Institute)**
2. **http://www.nccam.nih.gov/ (The National Institutes for Health, Office of Alternative and Complementary Medicine)**
3. **http://www.amtamassage.org (The American Massage Therapy Association)**
4. **http://www.upledger.com (The Upledger Institute Healthplex Center)**
5. **http://www.USABP.org (U.S. Association for Body Psychotherapy) http://EABP.org (European Association for Body Psychotherapy)**
6. **http://www.rubenfeldsynergy.com (Rubenfeld Synergy Method)**

CONGRATULATIONS!

You have finished all the chapters in this second book. You have completed some powerful, life-transforming exercises. You have self-reflected and contemplated how and why you touch and how you might benefit from therapy that includes talk and touch. Stories of individual revelations and transformations may have intrigued you and perked your curiosity. If you have gained personal insight, understanding of your self and others, and you want to continue on this path of loving and healing your life, then you will surely benefit from reading and following the exercises in the next two chapters in this valuable book.

MORE TO COME!

Love Me … Please

Love Me … Please, the first book in this four part series, leads us on a path toward loving … truly loving, from the center of our being. Love is the ultimate aphrodisiac. Love is patient, kind, unyielding, enduring and steadfast. Love overcomes all obstacles. But what most of us have called love, our human concepts and human attempts at love, with its sense of limited supply, ownership, and "what's in it for me" attitude, is filled with illusion, self-consciousness, insecurity, doubt and emotional upheaval. True love, unconditional love, a higher state of love, is limitless, boundless, and the ultimate creative power of the universe.

This book is meant for lovers, people who love, people who want love, people who have loved, and people who want to love again. You will not find simplistic answers and easy to follow formulas for creating love. You will have to look deep into your own consciousness – your thoughts, beliefs, attitudes, memories and dreams – to find the love, the fullest love, that you can bring into your life. And you will be reminded, over and over, to bring that love back to your own self so that you can fully share your loving self with others.

Heal Me … Please

Healing happens in every moment, in every cell and organ of our body. Loving, touching, and being touched with love, we heal. When we heal, our bodies relax and our lives come into balance. In healing, we discover our own truth, face our inner spirit, and we begin to know our connection to a higher source. In ***Heal Me … Please,*** the 4th book in the series, we examine the healing process: what we believe about healing, how we have healed our self and others, and how we can create healing in our bodies, our intimate relationships, our sexuality, and our lives.

Sexual and Spiritual Reawakening

We are all sexual beings. Sexuality teaches. Sexuality heals. Sometimes our sexuality hurts. When we allow our hearts to feel love and our bodies to feel pleasure, we are sexual. Being sexual is being alive. Feeling our sexual aliveness reawakens us to who we are. By allowing full sexual expression into our life, we cannot help but discover our spiritual nature.

We are all spiritual beings. Connecting to our spiritual nature and spiritual potential brings us an accepting appreciation of life. The path of discovering our spiritual connection can be difficult, painful and may reveal to us our deepest, darkest, most unloving personal attributes.

Our life path is a spiritual path, the process of rediscovering our connection to all that is. No matter which direction we choose to take, all paths will eventually lead us home. Every spiritual teaching reminds us of that simple truth. If we resist knowing this truth and pursue a self-centered and purely material way of life, we may encounter more struggle, more difficulties, and more tests than necessary. But even if we do pursue a spiritual path, there are still obstacles and difficulties to be overcome. The difference is that knowing our spiritual essence provides emotional strength and calmness in the face of any stormy life issues, problems and concerns.

Sexual and Spiritual Reawakening is a simple guide to help you live a more fulfilling, life affirming and joyful existence.

Have any of the words or exercises in this book touched a sensitive place in your thoughts, emotions or beliefs?

Are you ready to Lose

- **Your fears?**
- **Your doubts?**

Are you ready to Create

- **Love and healing?**

It's NOT Too Late!

NOW IS THE TIME TO CREATE HEALING AND LOVE IN YOUR LIFE!

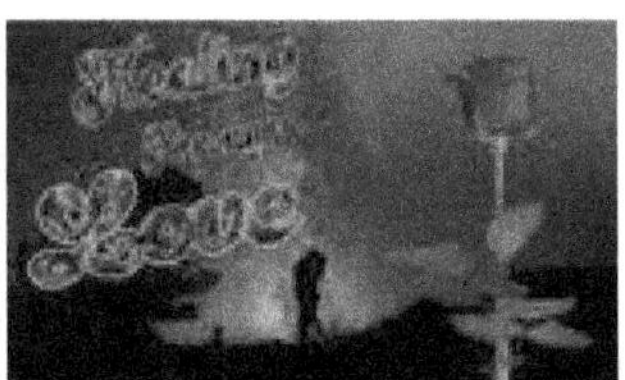

LoveNow.life/HealingThroughLoveSession

ALSO BY DR. ERICA GOODSTONE

KINDLE BOOKS

Beautiful Bare Feet: Fetish or Fantasy
Be Who You Are: The Greatest Gift of All
The Delicate Dance of Love
Your Body Believes You
It's a Sensational World
Touching Matters - The Profound Effects of Body Therapy
Let All Your Senses Speak – As You Heal
Touching Stories
Ordinary People, Ordinary Yet Extraordinary Sex
Sexual Reawakening: 10 Simple Steps
Sexual and Spiritual Reawakening – At Last!
The Science Of Being Well - Wallace D. Wattles author,
Annotated and Illustrated by Dr. Erica Goodstone
The Science Of Getting Rich **- Wallace D. Wattles author,**
Annotated and Illustrated by Dr. Erica Goodstone

Books and EBooks are available at
Amazon.com, Smashwords.com and Lulu.com

DIGITAL PROGRAMS

Love Touch Heal Video Series
Healing Through Love Audio Series
Love Lessons For Your Soul
Love Touch Heal Relationship Program

VIRTUAL SUMMITS

Men and Love Series
Women and Love Summit
Sexual Reawakening Summit

Love Me Touch Me Heal Me Summit
Healing Recovery Retreat
Miraculous Healing Master Class Summit
Science And Poetry of Love Summit
The Science of Being Well Docuseries

Programs, courses and summits available at https://DrEricaGoodstone.com

AMAZON REVIEWS

If you have enjoyed reading this book, please consider leaving an Amazon review. The author will be most grateful because this enables her to reach more people who want to create more love in their lives.

www.ingramcontent.com/pod-product-compliance
Lightning Source LLC
Chambersburg PA
CBHW080334270326
41927CB00014B/3211